Cambridge Medical Reviews

Neurobiology and Psychiatry   Volume 2

T0297307

Cambridge Medical Reviews set out to provide regular volumes of critically selected review material in a growing range of emerging and established disciplines within clinical medicine. They will concentrate particularly on areas where advances in basic biomedical science have a substantial contribution to make to the understanding and treatment of disease.

Rigorous standards of selection and editing ensure a reliable, topical and clinically relevant series of volumes, focused to meet the requirements of clinicians and research workers in each discipline.

Neurobiology and Psychiatry

Editor

Robert Kerwin
Institute of Psychiatry, University of London, London, UK

Advisory editors

David Dawbarn
Department of Medicine, Bristol Royal Infirmary, Bristol, UK

James McCulloch
Wellcome Surgical Institute and Hugh Fraser Neuroscience Laboratories, University of Glasgow, Glasgow, UK

Carol Tamminga
Inpatient Program, Maryland Psychiatry Research Center, Baltimore, Maryland, USA

Contents of Volume I

Cambridge Medical Reviews

Neurobiology and Psychiatry
Volume 2

EDITOR

ROBERT KERWIN
Institute of Psychiatry, University of London, London, UK

ADVISORY EDITORS

DAVID DAWBARN
Department of Medicine, Bristol Royal Infirmary, Bristol, UK

JAMES McCULLOCH
Wellcome Surgical Institute and Hugh Fraser Neuroscience Laboratories,
University of Glasgow, Glasgow, UK

CAROL TAMMINGA
Inpatient Program, Maryland Psychiatric Research Center, Baltimore, Maryland, USA

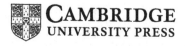

CAMBRIDGE
UNIVERSITY PRESS

CAMBRIDGE UNIVERSITY PRESS
Cambridge, New York, Melbourne, Madrid, Cape Town,
Singapore, São Paulo, Delhi, Tokyo, Mexico City

Cambridge University Press
The Edinburgh Building, Cambridge CB2 8RU, UK

Published in the United States of America by Cambridge University Press, New York

www.cambridge.org
Information on this title: www.cambridge.org/9780521203517

First published 1993
First paperback edition 2011

A catalogue record for this publication is available from the British Library

ISBN 978-0-521-43483-6 Hardback
ISBN 978-0-521-20351-7 Paperback
Additional resources for this publication at www.cambridge.org/9780521203517

Contents

Contributors

ALLEN, S J, Department of Medicine (Care of the Elderly), Bristol Royal Infirmary, Bristol BS2 8HW, UK

BEARN, J A, Section of Studies of Addiction, Institute of Psychiatry, De Crespigny Park, London SE5 8AF, UK

BOGERTS, B, Histological Laboratories, Department of Psychiatry, Rheinische Landesklinik, University of Düsseldorf, Bergische Landstrasse, 4000 Düsseldorf, Germany

DAWBARN, D, Department of Medicine (Care of the Elderly), Bristol Royal Infirmary, Bristol BS2 8HW, UK

EVERALL, I P, Institute of Psychiatry, De Crespigny Park, London SE5 8AF, UK

FALKAI, P, Histological Laboratories, Department of Psychiatry, Rheinische Landesklinik, University of Düsseldorf, Bergische Landstrasse, 4000 Düsseldorf, Germany

GALLO, J-M, Department of Neurology, Institute of Neurology, Institute of Psychiatry, De Crespigny Park, London SE5 8AF, UK

GILL, M, Section of Genetics, Institute of Psychiatry, De Crespigny Park, London SE5 8AF, UK

HARDY J, Department of Biochemistry, St Mary's Medical School, Norfolk Place, Praed Street, London WC1, UK

HOLLAND, A J, Institute of Psychiatry, De Crespigny Park, London SE5 8AF, UK

HONER, W G, Department of Psychiatry, University of British Columbia, Jack Bell Research Centre, 2660 Oak Street, Vancouver BC, Canada V6K 2Z6

KENNEDY, J I, Department of Psychiatry, University of Toronto, Toronto, Canada

KESHAVAN, M S, Department of Psychiatry, Western Psychiatric Institute, 3811 O'Hara Street, Pittsburgh PA 15213, USA

LANTOS, P L, Department of Neuropathology, De Crespigny Park, London SE5 8AF, UK

MacGOWAN, S H, Department of Medicine (Care of the Elderly), Bristol Royal Infirmary, Bristol BS2 8HW, UK

PETTEGREW, J W, Department of Psychiatry, Western Psychiatric Institute, 3811 O'Hara Street, Pittsburgh PA 15213, USA

Contributors

RAVEN, P W, Department of Psychiatry, Institute of Psychiatry, De Crespigny Park, London SE5 8AF, UK
WALSH, C, Section of Genetics, Institute of Psychiatry, De Crespigny Park, London SE5 8AF, UK

Preface

The second in this series of Cambridge Medical Reviews in Neurobiology and Psychiatry, there is much still to cover in the area of schizophrenia and Alzheimer's disease as well as new advances in molecular genetics, developmental biology and new imaging technology and this volume attempts to keep abreast with all these developments. Again, the aim is to review *in depth* areas of real progress rather than a broad superficial sweep and it is this aim which dominates the choice of topics. Similarly, as in volume 1 the authors are chosen for their youth and expertise, such that they are still very much hands on in their research as well as being internationally recognised. This is to ensure the best technical quality of these reviews.

It is planned that Volume 3 will be devoted to recent advances in neuroimaging technology in psychiatric research. In the meantime, I would like to thank Richard Barling and Jocelyn Foster at CUP for ensuring continuity of the series.

Robert Kerwin
Institute of Pyschiatry

Molecular genetics and the major psychoses

M GILL and C WALSH

The hypothesis that the major psychoses, schizophrenia and manic depression, are largely genetic disorders is supported by an impressive body of data. What remains in question is the extent and mode of transmission of that genetic contribution, which genes are involved, and how DNA mutations might interact with the environment to produce the constellation of symptoms known as schizophrenia and manic depression.

Defining the phenotype

Defining the phenotype for genetic study presents a number of problems for the major psychoses. First, diagnoses which depend on the identification and assessment of diverse groups of clinical symptoms may not define discrete phenotypes in the genetic sense, and what is considered a clinically homogenous entity may in fact represent several disorders of distinct etiology. Indeed, in the case of schizophrenia, a number of subtypes have been proposed which, if valid, are likely to differ in the extent to which genetic and environmental factors contribute to their etiology[1,2].

Secondly, it is not clear which related diagnoses should be included in the phenotypic definition. In the case of schizophrenia, family studies have shown that non psychotic diagnoses such as schizotypal or paranoid personality disorder cluster within the families of schizophrenic probands (for review see Leviston and Mowry[3]). It is likely, therefore, that these 'spectrum disorders' are genetically related to schizophrenia and may represent a modified expression of the same disease gene or genes. A similar situation arises in the case of major depression and cyclothymic personality in relation to manic depression. However, the specificity with which these disorders represent the phenotype is low. Further doubt arises with regard to the status of schizoaffective disorder, found in families of both schizophrenia and bipolar probands. On the basis of this observation, it has been suggested that the two disorders are not distinct from each other, but rather that they occupy polar

All correspondence to: Dr M Gill, Genetics Section, Institute of Psychiatry, De Crespigny Park, Denmark Hill, London SE5 8AF, UK.

Cambridge Medical Reviews: Neurobiology and Psychiatry Volume 2
© Cambridge University Press

positions on a disease continuum. The decision as to where the phenotypic boundary exists may therefore be an arbitrary exercise, but have serious implications for the interpretation of genetic studies.

Finally, there is a large literature describing how the major psychoses can be mimicked by organic conditions[4-6]. The exact prevalence of such 'phenocopies' is unknown; however, one study[7] identified underlying organic pathology in as many as 6% of patients with 'functional' psychoses.

Genetic investigations of the psychoses would be considerably enhanced by the identification of stable biological markers or 'endophenotypes' which distinguish etiologically homogenous forms of disorder. Various neuropsychological and neurophysiological measures, eg smooth eye pursuit movements[8], have been proposed but none is, as yet, generally applicable.

Clinical genetics of the major psychoses
Since the early 1900s, family studies have consistently shown that schizophrenia clusters within families[9,10]. In addition, morbid risk is found to correlate with genetic proximity to an affected individual. A 10% lifetime risk of developing schizophrenia in first degree relatives, and a 3% risk in second degree relatives, contrasts with a risk of 1% in the general population[10]. Adoption studies indicate that this increased liability is the result of shared genes and not shared environment[11,12]. Furthermore, pooled data from twin studies demonstrate illness concordance rates of 53% in genetically identical monozygotic twins in contrast to 15% in dizygotic pairs[13].

Recent work suggests the possibility that environmental hazards are of greater relevance to the development of schizophrenia in young males whilst genetic factors may be of greater importance in females[14-16]. Variables other than gender may also influence risk. For example, some studies show that early onset in schizophrenic probands is associated with greater morbidity in relatives[16], although this is not a consistent finding[17]. This may suggest that age of onset and liability to develop schizophrenia are associated. Alternatively, it may indicate etiological heterogeneity, with families of early onset probands expressing a more highly genetic form of the disease.

Similar studies conducted for manic depression demonstrate a strong genetic influence in that disorder. An 8% lifetime risk of illness in relatives of manic depressive probands represents a marked increase above a population risk of 0.5%. Adoption studies support the genetic hypothesis as do twin studies, with MZ twins up to three times more likely to show illness concordance than DZ twin pairs[18].

Proposed modes of inheritance
In the case of Mendelian disorders such as Huntington's disease and cystic fibrosis, information regarding the mode of transmission is easily obtained from family data. The transmission of other disorders may resemble

Mendelian inheritance but with minor transgressions; a number of individuals with a disease genotype may fail to manifest the disorder (reduced penetrance) or some individuals may express the disorder in an attenuated form (variable expression).

In yet another group, genetic factors are known to be of etiological importance but there is no adherence or resemblance to Mendelian transmission. These are 'complex genetic disorders' and include such conditions as coronary heart disease, diabetes, many autoimmune disorders and the major psychoses. For these, the mode of inheritance is likely to be obscured by variable age of onset, reduced penetrance, nongenetic cases (phenocopies), environmental influences, unclear phenotypic boundaries and genetic heterogeneity.

Mathematical models of disease transmission

Mathematical models of disease transmission predict patterns of familial aggregation which can be tested against existing family data. This data may take the form of morbid risk figures for various classes of relatives (prevalence analysis), or consist of information on the segregation of illness within entire pedigrees (segregation analysis)[19]. In general, segregation analysis is favoured for its greater statistical power.

If values predicted by a model are significantly different from observed findings, the model does not fit, and is rejected. A more problematic and not uncommon situation arises when several models are equally acceptable, each providing a moderate fit. Models considered in this manner, some of which incorporate a liability threshold construct[20], include the generalized single major locus (GSL) and the multifactorial threshold (MFT) models. For the GSL model, liability to develop a disorder is conferred by a single gene whose penetrance can take any value between 0 and 1. In contrast, liability in the MFT model is determined by both polygenes and environmental factors. The GSL and MFT models are not mutually exclusive and a 'mixed' model has been proposed[21] in which both major genes and polygenes play a role.

Genetic transmission of schizophrenia

Some studies have found compatibility between the GSL model and family data but nearly all noted an underprediction of MZ twin concordance[22-24]. Several other studies were able to reject the model outright[25-27]. Overall, existing evidence is strongly against a single gene effect when schizophrenia is treated as a unitary disease.

Many findings in schizophrenia are, however, more compatible with the MFT model. Morbid risk in relatives increases as a function of the number of affected individuals in the family. It also increases as a function of severity of illness in the proband; this is supported by twin studies which show higher concordance rates when the proband twin has a severe and chronic illness. In addition, most multifactorial/polygenic disorders occur with a lifetime risk of greater than 1 in 500[28].

Genetic transmission of manic depression

Family data do not consistently support any model of inheritance in manic depression[19]. Early family studies suggested X-linked dominant inheritance[29], demonstrating an excess of affected females and a deficit of father to son transmission. Risch and Baron[30] estimated that up to 30% of the manic depressive population might carry the putative disease gene on the X chromosome (based on linkage results). However, the concept of an X-linked subgroup remains controversial[31] and consistent evidence for autosomal dominant inheritance is also lacking.

Models of transmission: implications for molecular genetics

For the psychoses, as with other complex genetic disorders, there is an unclear relationship between phenotype and genotype, and Mendelian patterns of segregation are not normally observed within families. Undoubtedly, for some of these disorders, Mendelian traits remain to be recognized, having been obscured so far by genetic heterogeneity, late onset or variable penetrance. Whether this applies to the major psychoses remains to be seen.

On the other hand, the major psychoses may more closely resemble traits such as height and intelligence, both with large genetic components. Thus they would be due to the additive effects of many genes, each contributing a minor amount of the total genetic variance. Indeed, many animal behaviours, such as alcohol sensitivity, nest building and aggressiveness appear to be truly polygenic, in that repeated selected breeding of animals for such traits fail to divide them into two behavioural extremes[32]. If only one or two major genes were responsible for the genetic effects of these behaviours, the relevant alleles would be sorted into the high and low lines in a few generations.

Some traits and disorders, previously considered polygenic, are yielding single gene subtypes. Hypertension in rats, for example, can be caused by major genes[33], and a subtype of diabetes in humans is caused by a dominant mutation at the glucokinase gene[34]. Alzheimer's disease, previously considered polygenic, can be caused by single gene mutations, detected with the aid of linkage analysis.

Demonstrating single gene subtypes in many disorders has, however, depended on obvious candidate genes, animal models or clear clinical subdivisions. In diabetes, the mutation on chromosome 7 causes an early onset, noninsulin dependent form of disease[34]. Moreover, the definition of the phenotype is assisted by biochemical tests. In the case of Alzheimer's disease[35], early onset delineated a clinical subtype, and the association with Down's syndrome indicated chromosome 21. The absence of animal models or clinical subdivision for the major psychoses makes the researchers task considerably more difficult. However, recent discoveries in other complex genetic disorders suggest that for the major psychoses, etiological and genetic heterogeneity are to be expected. Under these circumstances clinical genetic studies and mathematical modelling of disease transmission are unlikely to indicate which molecular biological techniques are appropriate. A broad approach is therefore justified in preliminary investigations. The remainder of this chapter will discuss current molecular strategies and results to date.

The molecular genetics of the psychoses: candidate genes and gene finding techniques

A candidate gene is one for which there is some a priori reason to suspect its involvement in the etiology of the disorder in question. In the case of the major psychoses, there are many genes that fall into the category of 'possible candidates', but few, if any, that fall into the category of 'probable candidates'. Although all brain specific genes could be considered candidates for the major psychoses, choice of genes for study should be theory led. Thus the hypothesis that neurodevelopmental abnormality may lead to schizophrenia suggests a possible role for genes which determine or modify neurodevelopment processes[36].

In manic depression, as in schizophrenia, there is a range of etiological theories; one of these concerns cation transport. It has been suggested that, in normal controls, the enzyme Na+K+ATPase is increased in lymphocytes following incubation in lithium or ethacrynate[37]. This 'upregulation' is absent or attenuated in both euthymic drug-free manic depressive patients, and in those taking lithium. These results confirmed earlier work by Naylor and Smith[38]. The authors suggest that this altered response of the enzyme is an enduring trait marker in manic depression. The enzyme is composed of two subunits, a large catalytic subunit, and a smaller glycoprotein subunit. The catalytic subunit is encoded by at least three separate genes. All of these are potential candidate genes.

Once a particular gene is identified as a candidate, it remains to be assessed if, and to what degree, it contributes to the disease liability. Clarification of a particular gene's involvement can be approached in a number of ways: gene structure and function may be examined directly or, alternatively, the techniques of genetic linkage or association can be employed. One potential advantage of genetic linkage methods is that they can identify the location of abnormal genes without requiring prior knowledge of the disease process.

Candidate genes: functional analysis

Candidate genes may be studied directly, their structure and function compared between patients and controls. Functional abnormalities may occur anywhere from transcription of the gene into RNA, through processing of that RNA, to translation into a protein. The function of a gene is studied by examination of messenger RNA (mRNA). The relative site of action of the gene in the brain and the abundance of its expression is determined using in situ hybridization with cloned segments of transcribed gene. It is important to note, however, that the function of a set of genes may be disturbed as a secondary consequence of abnormality elsewhere.

For schizophrenia, one set of genes studied in this manner are those receptors stimulated by the excitatory neurotransmitter L-glutamate. This neurotransmitter provides the major afferent input to the hippocampus. Its receptors are divided pharmacologically into 5 classes; N-methyl-D-aspartate (NMDA), alpha-amino-3-hydroxy-5-methyl-4-isoxazole propionate (AMPA), kainate and 2-amino-4-phsophonobutyrate (AP4), known as ionotrophic receptors and one metabotrophic receptor (mGluR)[39]. In addition, there is evidence that alternative splicing of the mRNA occurs, thereby adding to receptor diversity[40]. Abnormalities in the binding of glutamate receptor ligands in the brains of schizophrenics have been reported and molecular studies are a natural progression from such findings[41]. Recently, Harrison et al.[42] have reported a decrease in mRNA encoding a non-NMDA glutamate receptor in hippocampal tissue from schizophrenic patients compared to normals. Whether this is specific, or part of a more widespread abnormality in gene expression they are unable to say. Nor has a secondary effect of medication been ruled out as an explanation.

Candidate genes: structural analysis
To date, there has been little work examining the structure of any particular candidate gene in patients. One study reported fully sequencing the functionally significant parts of the D2 receptor in 14 schizophrenic patients, but found no structural changes[43].

Gene finding techniques: genetic linkage and its application to the major psychoses
Genetic linkage refers to the observation that two genetic traits may be coinherited rather than independently inherited as Mendel prediction in his second law. If 2 genetic traits are caused by genes which exist close together on the same chromosome then during meiosis, recombination between them will occur only rarely, and they will be passed on to offspring together.

A genetic trait or a disease is the result of a genetic polymorphism; a base pair sequence difference between two homologous strands of DNA that can be detected. In the case of a disease or a trait, the genotypic difference is inferred from the phenotype. In the case of a DNA polymorphism, it is detected by direct examination of the DNA. DNA polymorphisms, or markers, are known throughout the genome, and their segregation in families can be determined and compared with the segregation of a genetic disease. If cosegregation is apparent, then the conclusion is that the disease gene is located close to the marker polymorphism.

The LOD (*L*og of the *odD*s ratio) score method of Morton is widely used in the assessment of linkage. It is a powerful method, based on the theory of likelihood, using all the information available within large pedigrees. For single gene disorders, a LOD score > 3 is taken as evidence of linkage, and a score of < −2 as evidence of exclusion of linkage; numbers in between are inconclusive.

The LOD score method requires the estimation of genetic parameters describing disease and marker transmission. The appropriate model and parameters are not known for the major psychoses, and the effects of misspecification on the reliability of the LOD score is not certain although such misspecification has been shown to decrease the power to detect, rather than to falsely infer, linkage[45].

The sib-pair method of Penrose[46], and its modern modifications[47,48] may be more robust to misspecification of genetic parameters, and are thought to offer an alternative to the LOD score method in complex genetic diseases. In the affected sib-pair method, if a disease and a genetic marker are truly unlinked then, in a large sample of affected sib-pairs, marker alleles will be shared and unshared in equal proportions. If alleles are shared significantly more than expected, then one conclusion is that linkage exists between marker and disease. With many highly polymorphic markers throughout the genome, 'significant' results will clearly occur by chance. Replication, as with LOD score results, will be essential.

In the major psychoses, the absence of a priori evidence for single gene subtypes and a reliable method of clinical subdivision causes difficulties for the linkage method of analysis. It remains at present no more than an article of faith whether or not single gene transmission exists in a significant proportion of families, multiply affected with one or other of the major psychoses.

Nevertheless, there are two reasons for using linkage analysis to search for genes of major effect. The first, as outlined above, is the evidence from other complex genetic traits that single gene subtypes may be much more common than has been considered to date. The second reason is the enormous potential for a serious breakthrough in our knowledge that may result from identification of such genes, even if mutations in them cause disease in only a minority of large multiply affected families.

It is the proven ability of molecular genetic techniques to facilitate significant advances in knowledge of pathophysiological mechanisms that caused such excitement when initial results in the case of the major psychoses were promising[49], and such disappointment when these results turned out to be false leads[50].

Linkage studies in schizophrenia: results to date

The casual reader in this subject would be forgiven if he thought that linkage studies in schizophrenia began with chromosome 5. One of the earliest studies showing promising results was a study of HLA genotypes in families multiply affected by 'schizotaxia': a broadly defined clinical phenotype including schizophrenia and schizotypal personality[51]. Four further studies failed to confirm these findings[52-55]. One study employed the affected sib-pair method along with the LOD score method of analysis[52]. Overall, the conclusion was that a 'dominant' gene for schizophrenia was unlikely to be located close to the HLA locus.

The advent of DNA markers provides a catalogue of polymorphic markers scattered throughout the genome. On the basis of a trisomy of part of chromosome 5q apparently cosegregating with schizophrenia in a small family[56], Sherrington et al.[57] examined the segregation of three DNA markers mapping to the region in five Icelandic and two British families. Evidence for linkage was found; it was strongest when a variety of disorders, some probably related to schizophrenia, and some not, were included in the analysis. The quoted maximum LOD score of 6.49 was generated using an extension of the method which allows data from a number of closely linked markers to be used simultaneously. This procedure, although safe for known single gene disorders, can falsely inflate the evidence for linkage and is not recommended for a preliminary analysis. The maximum LOD score between a marker and the disease in the study by Sherrington et al. was 3.96; strong but not conclusive evidence for linkage. Furthermore, if, as has been recommended by some observers[58,59], the maximum 2-point LOD score is corrected to take into account multiple genetic and diagnostic models, then the result would have been reduced by 1.38, ie 2.58.

Simultaneously, Kennedy et al.[60] failed to confirm the findings of Sherrington et al. using a large Swedish family. That this result could have been due to linkage heterogeneity was suggested by Kennedy et al.[60] and Lander[61]. Subsequently, however, five further studies have been reported[62-66] all of which found no evidence of linkage. Finally, the group that produced the initial promising findings have now extended their studies on chromosome 5q by generating new, highly polymorphic markers within the region. They have determined the genotypes at these markers of both the original families and a new collection. None of their recent results confirms previous findings, and, indeed, effectively excludes the region from containing a single gene of major effect in the etiology of schizophrenia[67].

There is no evidence of X-linkage in schizophrenia. However, a role for the sex chromosomes is suggested by findings of an excess of schizophrenia in individuals with sex chromosome aneuplodies and by the finding that pairs of affected relatives are more likely to be of the same, than opposite, sex[68,69].

Crow[70] suggested that these results could be explained if the gene(s) for schizophrenia was located in the pseudoautosomal region of the sex chromosomes. This is a small area located at the distal end of both the X and Y chromosome. It contains sequence homology between the X and Y chromosomes and exchange of genetic material takes place during meiosis. Depending on its position within the region, a gene may be transmitted in either a sex-linked or 'pseudoautosomal' manner. In their study of 83 sib-pairs affected with schizophrenia Collinge and colleagues[71] found tentative evidence of linkage to pseudoautosomal markers. However, because of the limited power of the affected sib-pair method, the authors concluded that examination of the hypothesis was required in a larger sample. A second group have also reported evidence of nonrandom segregation of marker alleles to affected sib-pairs[72]. Others[73], while detecting an excess of same sex sib-pairs, found no evidence for linkage in this region.

More recently, there has been some interest in the long arm of chromosome 11. Several families have been reported in which balanced translocations involving chromosome 11q apparently cosegregate with psychotic illness[74–76]. In addition, genes encoding the D2 receptor, porphobilinogen deaminase, and tyrosinase map to this region, and could be considered candidate genes for the schizophrenia. In a systematic search using a large sample of multiply affected pedigrees, Gill et al.[77] found little evidence suggesting the presence of a gene of major effect in this region.

Linkage studies in manic depression
Early linkage studies in manic depression have concentrated on two areas of the genome; the X-chromosome and the HLA region of chromosome 6. The interest in the X-chromosome began when Rosanoff et al.[78] proposed this form of transmission on the basis of their family and twin studies. A number of early studies showed apparent cosegregation (linkage) between the X-linked genetic markers, colour blindness and G6PD[29,79]. Evidence of linkage to the blood group marker Xg was also found[80]. As these two markers are on opposite ends of the X-chromosome linkage to both in the same pedigrees is unlikely. Mendlewicz and Fleiss[81] studied both markers and concluded that a putative X-linked bipolar gene was situated between the markers. Their evidence for colour blindness linkage was stronger than that for Xg. Many further studies ensued, most demonstrating evidence of varying degrees in favour of linkage[82–85], but some showing evidence against X-linkage[86,87]. Detailed analysis of the pedigrees studied by Baron et al.[85] suggest that the LOD scores are robust to a variety of phenotype definitions and to variations in genetic parameters[88]. These authors suggest that the X-linked form of manic depression is characterized by severity, early age of onset, high familial prevalence of the bipolar phenotype and high recurrence rate of major depression.

There have also been reports of linkage to factor IX[89]. These genes are some distance apart, and linkage to both may not be compatible, thus raising the possibility of two X-linked genes or false positive results at one or other locus.

In affective disorders, there appears to have been no good reason to study HLA antigens other than their presence and extreme variability, and thus suitability as linkage markers. In 1981, Weitkamp et al.[94] reported that affected sibling pairs shared HLA haplotypes more often than would be expected by chance. A previous study had reported similar findings[90]. Further studies[91-93] failed to confirm these findings and cast doubt on the validity of the statistical methods of Weitkamp et al.[94].

Evidence for a susceptibility locus close to the tyrosine hydroxylase gene on chromosome 11 in a large Amish pedigree[95] was reported, but was not supported by studies of other pedigrees[96-98]. This was initially interpreted as evidence of genetic heterogeneity, but reanalysis and extension of the Amish pedigree led to a drop in the LOD score, thus casting doubt on the original report[99].

Genetic association and its use in the major psychoses

At present, there is no obvious method of subdividing the major psychoses such that one or more subdivisions are more likely (a) to be etiologically homogeneous or (b) to demonstrate Mendelian transmission. Applying linkage methods to the whole may fail if there is significant etiological or genetic heterogeneity. An alternative method of genetic analysis, less dependent on the underlying disease model, is to test for association between particular alleles of a polymorphism and the disease phenotype. This method requires a large sample of unrelated affected individuals and has been successful for HLA-associated diseases[100], for diseases associated with red blood cell surface antigens[101] and for heart disease[102]. DNA polymorphisms have greatly expanded the scope of these studies, and are available within, or close to, any gene of interest.

Genetic association is thought to arise as follows. If a mutation contributes to a disease then, clearly, it will occur more frequently in patients than controls. However, closely surrounding DNA will also tend to occur more frequently in patients. If, within this surrounding region, there is another polymorphism then certain alleles at that polymorphism will also occur more frequently in patients than controls. This phenomenon, also known as linkage disequilibrium, is often detected between DNA markers from the same location[103], and is very common between HLA classes. Whether two polymorphisms are indeed in linkage disequilibrium depends on the period of time since both polymorphisms arose, the distance between them and the frequency of recombination in the region.

Ferns et al.[104] describe DNA polymorphisms within or near genes as simply markers which may or may not be in linkage disequilibrium with gene variations (mutations) that may predispose to disease. Sobell et al.[105] point out that the strategy of testing markers within or near genes for evidence of allelic association with the disease phenotype depends on the presence of linkage disequilibrium between the causative mutation and an allele of the polymorphism, and that there are many reasons why this may not exist. She suggests examining only DNA polymorphisms that are a sequence variation affecting protein structure or expression. Both general association studies and the variant described by Sobell are, for practical purposes, confined to candidate genes. If one, or a few, candidate genes were strongly implicated in the major psychoses then the later strategy is to be preferred. However, it cannot be considered a screening method. With due attention to statistical methodology and choice of polymorphisms, genetic association studies can be used to efficiently screen a large number of 'possible' candidate genes.

The ready availability of HLA genotypes, and the known negative association of schizophrenia with rheumatoid arthritis[106] has resulted in a large number of studies examining the distribution of HLA alleles in schizophrenia. McGuffin and Sturt[107] outline 14 studies with significant differences in various allele frequencies between schizophrenics and controls. All except 1 allele, HLA A9, appear to be inconsistent between studies. A number of studies reported significantly increased frequency of HLA A9 in schizophrenics compared with controls. Two studies, however, reported HLA A9 to be significantly less frequent than in controls. Allowing for multiple testing (multiple alleles)[107] McGuffin and Sturt conclude that the combined chi-square for the A9 association remains strongly significant.

More recently, using DNA markers at the porphobilinogen deaminase (PBGD) gene, Sanders et al.[108] reported one allele to be significantly associated with the disease phenotype. Studies by Owen et al.[109] and Nimgaonker et al.[110] have subsequently failed to confirm this finding. Owen and colleagues calculate that their study had a power greater than 90% to detect an effect of the magnitude of that reported by Sanders et al.[108].

In affective disorders, some attention has been given to the tyrosine hydroxylase gene on chromosome 11p. This gene maps close to the markers used in the Amish and subsequent linkage studies on chromosome 11p. Tyrosine hydroxylase is the rate limiting enzyme in catecholamine synthesis, and can therefore be considered a candidate gene. Todd and O'Malley[111] reported the frequency of alleles from 2 RFLPs in 18 patients and controls and found no differences. Leboyer et al.[112], however, found strongly significant associations between RFLPs at both ends of the gene using a sample of 50 bipolar patients and matched controls. Korner et al.[113] and Gill et al.[114] failed to confirm the finding in similar size patient samples, but Gill et al. pointed out that one of the polymorphisms demonstrates a similar, but nonsignificant, distribution in both negative studies. The heterogeneity chi-square statistic of Woolf[115] was not significant allowing the studies to be pooled. Combined evidence suggests an association ($p < 0.02$) between the polymorphism and bipolar disorder. The odds ratio was 1.5 with 95% confidence intervals of 1.1–2.1.

M Gill and C Walsh

Conclusions

There is not yet a 'molecular biology' of the major psychoses, although research efforts to understand the nature of the genetic predisposition rely heavily on molecular biological techniques. None the less, necessary components of future research of this kind are clinical genetic studies. These will improve definition of the phenotype and may identify 'endophenotypes', more relevant to laboratory analyses.

Although genetic linkage and association studies have not yet clearly identified novel candidate genes or chromosome regions, some interesting findings remain to be confirmed or refuted such as the involvement of the HLA region, or the proposed pseudoautosomal locus in schizophrenia, proposed X-linkage in manic depression and association with tyrosine hydroxylase marker alleles. Methods of analysis and awareness of pitfalls have improved allowing optimism for the future. In situ hybridization will be used to study the function of genes such as those encoding glutamate receptor subunits. And, finally, direct DNA sequencing will determine the structure of the most likely candidate genes in patients and controls. In time, DNA mutations will be identified and their role in the etiology of the major psychoses elucidated.

References

(1) Castle D, Murray RM. The neurodevelopmental basis of sex differences in schizophrenia. *Psych Med* 1991; 21: 565–75.
(2) Murray RM, O'Callaghan E, Castle D et al. A neurodevelopmental approach to the classification of schizophrenia. *Schiz Bull*; in press.
(3) Leviston DF, Mowry BJ. Defining the schizophrenia spectrum: issues for genetic linkage studies. *Schiz Bull* 1991; 17: 491–514.
(4) Davison K, Bagley CR. Schizophrenia-like psychoses associated with organic disorders of the central nervous system: a review of the literature. In: Herrington RN, ed. *Current problems in neuropsychiatry*. Ashford, Kent: Headley Brothers, 1969.
(5) Krauthammer C, Klerman GL. Secondary mania. *Arch Gen Psych* 1978; 35: 1333–9.
(6) Propping P. Genetic disorders presenting as 'schizophrenia'. Karl Bonhoeffer's early view of the psychoses in the light of medical genetics. *Hum Genet* 1983; 65: 1–10.
(7) Johnston EC, Cooling NJ, Frith CD et al. Phenomenology of the organic and functional psychoses and the overlap between them. *Br J Psych* 1988; 153: 770–6.
(8) Blackwood D, StClair D, Muir W et al. Auditory P300 and eye tracking dysfunction in schizophrenic pedigrees. *Arch Gen Psych* 1991; 48: 899–909.
(9) Rudin E. *Zur vererbung und neuentstehung der Dementia Praecox*. Berlin: Springer, 1916.
(10) Gottesman II. *Schizophrenia genesis: the origins of madness*. New York: WH Freeman, 1991: 95–7.

(11) Heston LL. The genetics of schizophrenia and schizoid disease. *Science* 1970; 167: 249–56.
(12) Kety SS, Rosenthal D, Wender PH et al. The biological and adoptive families of individuals who became schizophrenic: prevalence of mental illness and other characteristics. In: *The nature of schizophrenia: new approaches to research and treatment*, Wynne LC, Cromwell RL, Matthysse S, eds. New York: Wiley, 1978.
(13) Kendler KS. Overview: a current perspective on twin studies of schizophrenia. *Am J Psych* 1983; 140: 1413–25.
(14) Bellodi L, Bussoleni C, Scorza-Smeraldi R et al. Family study of schizophrenia: exploratory analysis for relevant factors. *Schiz Bull* 1986; 12: 120–8.
(15) Goldstein JM, Tsuang MT, Farrone SV. Gender and schizophrenia: implications for understanding the heterogeneity of the illness. *J Psych Res* 1989; 28: 243–53.
(16) Sham P, Jones P, Foerster A et al. Age at onset, gender, and the familial occurrence of schizophrenia: evidence for aetiological heterogeneity. *Br J Psych*; in press.
(17) Kendler KS, Tsuang MT, Hays P. Age at onset in schizophrenia. *Arch Gen Psych* 1987; 44: 881–90.
(18) McGuffin P, Katz R, Bebbington P. Hazard, heredity, and depression: a family study. *J Psych Res* 1987; 21: 365–75.
(19) Faraone SV, Tsuang MT. In: *The genetics of mood disorders*. Baltimore: The Johns Hopkins University Press, 1990.
(20) Falconer DS. The inheritance of liability to certain diseases, estimated from the incidence among relatives. *Ann Hum Genet* 1965; 29: 51–76.
(21) Meehl PE. Specific genetic etiology, psychodynamics, and therapeutic nihilism. *Int J Ment Health* 1972; 1: 10–27.
(22) Elston RC, Campbell MA. Schizophrenia: evidence for a major gene hypothesis. *Behav Genet* 1970; 1: 3–10.
(23) Matthysse SW, Kidd KK. Estimating the genetic contribution to schizophrenia. *Am J Psych* 1976: 133: 185–191.
(24) Kidd KK, Cavalli-Sforza LL. An analysis of the genetics of schizophrenia. *Soc Biol* 1973; 20: 254–65.
(25) Baron M. Genetic models of schizophrenia. *Acta Psych Scand* 1982; 65: 263–75.
(26) O'Rourke DH, Gottesman II, Suarez BK et al. Refutation of the general single-locus model for the aetiology of schizophrenia. *Am J Hum Genet* 1982; 34: 325–33.
(27) McGue M, Gottesman II, Rao DC. Resolving genetic models for the transmission of schizophrenia. *Genet Epidem* 1985; 2: 99–110.
(28) Kendler KS. Familial aggregation of schizophrenia and schizophrenia spectrum disorders. *Arch Gen Psychiat* 1988; 45: 377–83.
(29) Reich T, Clayton PJ, Winokur G. Family history studies V. The genetics of mania. *Am J Psych* 1969; 125: 1359–68.
(30) Risch N, Baron M. Assessing the role of X-linked inheritance in bipolar-related major affective disorder. *J Psych Res* 1986; 20: 275–88.
(31) Hebebrand J. A critical appraisal of X-linked bipolar illness: evidence for the assumed mode of inheritance is lacking. *Br J Psychiat* 1992; 160: 7–11.

(32) Plomin R. The role of inheritance in behavior. *Science* 1990; 248: 183–8.

(33) Jacob HJ, Lindpainter K, Lincoln SE. Genetic mapping of a gene causing hypertension in the stroke-prone spontaneously hypertensive rat. *Cell* 191; 67: 213–24.

(34) Froguel Ph, Vaxillaire M, Sun F et al. Close linkage of glucokinase locus on chromosome 7p to early onset non-insulin-dependent diabetes mellitus. *Nature* 1992; 356: 162–4.

(35) Heyman A, Wilkinson WE, Stafford JA et al. Alzheimer's disease: a study of epidemiological aspects. *Ann Neurol* 1984; 15: 335–41.

(36) Jones P, Murray RM. The genetics of schizophrenia is the genetics of neuro-development. *Br J Psych* 1992; 158: 615–23.

(37) Wood AJ, Smith CE, Clarke EE et al. Altered in vitro adaptive responses of lymphocyte Na+K+ATPase in patients with manic-depressive psychosis. *J Affect Dis* 1991; 21: 199–206.

(38) Naylor GJ, Smith AH. Defective genetic control of sodium pump density in manic-depressive psychosis. *Psych Med* 1981; 11: 257–63.

(39) Masu M, Tanabe Y, Tsuchida K et al. Sequence and expression of a metabotropic glutamate receptor. *Nature* 1991; 349: 760–5.

(40) Sommer B, Keinanen K, Verdoorn TA et al. Flip and Flop: a cell-specific functional switch in glutamate-operated channels of the CNS. *Science* 1990; 249: 1580–5.

(41) Deakin JFW, Slater P, Simpson MDC et al. Frontal cortical and left temporal glutamatergic dysfunction in schizophrenia. *J Neurochem* 1989; 52: 1781–6.

(42) Harrison PJ, McLaughlin D, Kerwin RW. Decreased hippocampal expression of a glutamate receptor gene in schizophrenia. *Lancet* 1991; 337: 450–2.

(43) Sarker G, Kapelner S, Grandy DK et al. Direct sequencing of the dopamine D2 receptor (DRD2) in schizophrenics reveals three polymorphisms but no structural change in the receptor. *Genomics*; in press.

(44) Morton NE. Sequential tests for the detection of linkage. *Am J Hum Genet* 1955; 7: 277–318.

(45) Clerget-Darpoux F, Bonaiti-Pellie C, Hochez J. Effects of misspecifying genetic parameters in lod score analysis. *Biometrics* 1986; 42: 393–9.

(46) Penrose L. The general purpose sib-pair test. *Ann Eugenics* 1953; 6: 133–8.

(47) Suarez BK, Rice J, Reich T. The generalised sib-pair IBD distribution: its use in the detection of linkage. *Ann Hum Genet* 1978; 42: 87–94.

(48) Thompson G. Determining the mode of inheritance of RFLP-associated diseases using the affected sib-pair method. *Am J Hum Genet* 1986; 39: 207–21.

(49) Mullan M, Murray RM. The impact of molecular genetics on our understanding of the psychoses. *Br J Psych* 1989; 154: 591–5.

(50) Watt D, Edwards G. Doubt about evidence for a schizophrenia gene on chromosome 5. *Psych Med* 1991; 21: 279–85.

(51) Turner WJ. Genetic markers for schizophrenia. *Biol Psych* 1979; 14: 177–205.

(52) McGuffin P, Festenstein H, Murray RM. A family study of HLA antigens and other genetic markers in schizophrenia. *Psych Med* 1983; 13: 31–43.

(53) Chadda R, Kullhara P, Singh T et al. HLA antigens in schizophrenia: a family study. *Br J Psych* 1986; 149: 612–5.

(54) Goldin LR, DeLisi LF, Gershon ES. The relationship of HLA to schizophrenia in 10 nuclear families. *Psychiat Res* 1987; 20: 69–78.

(55) Andrews B, Watt DC, Gillespie C, Chapel H. A study of genetic linkage in schizophrenia. *Psych Med* 1987; 17: 363–70.

(56) Bassett AS, Jones BD, McGillivray BC, Pantzar JT. Partial trisomy chromosome 5 cosegregating with schizophrenia. *Lancet* 1988; 2: 799–801.

(57) Sherrington R, Brynjolffson J, Petursson H et al. Localization of a susceptibility locus for schizophrenia on chromosome 5. *Nature* 1988; 336: 164–7.

(58) Edwards JH, Watt DC. Caution in locating the gene(s) for affective disorder. *Psych Med* 1989; 19: 273–5.

(59) Risch N. A note on multiple testing procedures in linkage analysis. *Am J Hum Genet* 1991; 48: 1058–64.

(60) Kennedy JL, Giuffra LA, Moises HW et al. Evidence against linkage of schizophrenia to markers on chromosome 5 in a northern Swedish pedigree. *Nature* 1988; 336: 167–9.

(61) Lander ES. Splitting schizophrenia. *Nature* 1988; 336: 105–6.

(62) StClair D, Blackwood D, Muir W et al. No linkage of chromosome 5q11–q13 markers to schizophrenia in Scottish families. *Nature* 1989; 339: 305–9.

(63) Crowe RR, Black DW, Andreasen N et al. The Iowa multiplex family study of schizophrenia: linkage analysis on chromosome 5. *Eur Arch Psych Neurol Sci* 1990; 239: 290–2.

(64) Detera-Wadleigh S, Goldin L, Sherrington R et al. Exclusion of linkage to 5q11–13 in families with schizophrenia and other psychiatric disorders. *Nature* 1989; 340: 391–3.

(65) Aschauer H, Aschauer-Treiber G, Isenberg K et al. No evidence for linkage between chromosome 5 markers and schizophrenia. *Hum Hered* 1990; 40: 109–15.

(66) McGuffin P, Sargeant M, Hett G et al. Exclusion of a schizophrenia susceptibility gene from the chromosome 5q11–q13 region. New data and a reanalysis of previous reports. *Am J Hum Genet* 1990; 47: 524–32.

(67) Mankoo B, Sherrington R, Brynjolffson J et al. New microsatellite polymorphisms provide a highly polymorphic map of chromosome 5 bands q11.2–q13.3 for linkage analysis of Icelandic and English families affected by schizophrenia. *Psychiat Genet* 1991; 2: 17.

(68) Penrose LS. Auxillary genes for determining sex as contributory causes of mental illness. *J Ment Sci* 1942; 88: 308–16.

(69) Crowe RR, Black DW, Andreasen NC et al. The Iowa multiplex family study of schizophrenia: linkage analysis on chromosome 5. *Euro Arch Psych Neuro Sci* 1990; 239: 290–2.

(70) Crow TJ. Sex chromosomes and psychosis: the case for a pseudoautosomal locus. *Br J Psych* 1988; 153: 675–83.

(71) Collinge JS, DeLisis LD, Boccio A et al. Evidence for a pseudoautosomal locus for schizophrenia using the affected sibling pair method. *Br J Psych* 1991; 4: 624–9.

(72) d'Amato T, Campion D, Gorwood P et al. A pseudoautosomal locus in schizophrenia. *Br J Psych*; in press.

M Gill and C Walsh

(73) Asherson P, Parfitt E, Sargeant M et al. No evidence for a pseudo-autosomal locus for schizophrenia from linkage analysis of multiply affected families. *Br J Psych*; in press.
(74) StClair D, Blackwood D, Muir W et al. Association within a family of a balanced autosomal translocation with major mental illness. *Lancet* 1990; 336: 13–16.
(75) Smith M, Wasmuth J, McPherson JD et al. Cosegregation of an 11q22–9p22 translocation with affective disorder: proximity of the dopamine D2 receptor gene relative to the translocation breakpoint. *Am J Hum Genet* 1989; 45: 220.
(76) Holland A, Gosden C. A balanced chromosomal translocation partially co-segregating with psychotic illness in a family. *Psychiat Res* 1990; 32: 1–8.
(77) Gill M, Castle D, Hunt N et al. Tyrosine hydroxylase polymorphisms and bipolar affective disorder. *J Psych Res* 1991; 25: 179–84.
(78) Rosanoff AJ, Handy L, Plesset IR. The aetiology of manic-depressive syndromes with special references to their occurrence in twins. *Am J Psych* 1935; 91: 725–40.
(79) Mendlewicz J, Fleiss JL, Fieve RR. Evidence for X-linkage in the transmission of manic-depressive illness. *JAMA* 1973; 222: 1624–7.
(80) Winokur G, Tanna VL. Possible role of X-linked dominant factor in manic-depressive diseases. *Dis Nerv Sys* 1969; 30: 89–93.
(81) Mendlewicz J, Fleiss JL. Linkage studies with X-chromosome markers in bipolar (manic-depression) and unipolar (depressive) illnesses. *Biol Psych* 1974; 9: 261–94.
(82) Baron M. Linkage between an X-chromosome marker (deutan color blindness) and bipolar affective illness. *Arch Gen Psych* 1977; 34: 721–5.
(83) Mendlewicz J, Linkowski P, Guroff JJ. Color blindness linkage to manic-depressive illness. *Arch Gen Psych* 1979; 36: 1442–7.
(84) DelZompo M, Bochetta A, Goldin LR. Linkage between X-chromosome markers and manic depressive illness: two Sardinian pedigrees. *Act Psych Scand* 1984; 70: 282–7.
(85) Baron M, Risch N, Hamburger R et al. Genetic linkage between x-chromosome markers and bipolar affective illness. *Nature* 1987; 326: 289–92.
(86) Gershon ES, Targum SD, Matthysse S et al. Color blindness not closely linked to bipolar illness. *Arch Gen Psych* 1979; 36: 1423–30.
(87) Berrettini WH, Goldin LR, Gelernter J et al. x-chromosome markers and manic-depressive illness: rejection of linkage in nine bipolar pedigrees. *Arch Gen Psych* 1990; 47: 366–73.
(88) Baron M, Hamburger R, Sandkuyl LA et al. The impact of phenotypic variation on genetic analysis: application to X-linkage in manic-depressive illness. *Act Psych Scand* 1990; 82: 196–203.
(89) Mendlewicz J, Simon P, Sevy S et al. Polymorphic DNA marker on X-chromosome and manic-depression. *Lancet* 1987; 1230–2.
(90) Smeraldi E, Negri F, Melica A et al. HLA system and affective disorders: a sibship genetic study. *Tissue Antigens* 1978; 12: 270.
(91) Mendlewicz J, Verbanck P, Linkowski P et al. (1981) HLA antigens in affective disorders and schizophrenia. *J Aff Dis* 1981; 3: 17–24.

(92) Suarez BK, Croughan J. Is the major histocompatibility complex linked to genes that increase susceptibility to affective disorder? A critical appraisal. *Psych Res* 1982; 7: 19–27.

(93) Goldin LR, Clerget-Darpoux F, Gershon ES. Relationship of HLA to major affective disorder not supported. *Psych Res* 19982; 7: 29–45.

(94) Weitkamp LR, Stancer HC, Persad E et al. Depressive disorders and HLA: a gene on chromosome 6 that can affect behavior. *N Eng J Med* 1981; 305: 1301–6.

(95) Egeland JA, Gerhard DS, Pauls DL et al. Bipolar affective disorders linked to DNA markers on chromosome 11. *Nature* 1987; 325: 783–7.

(96) Hodgkinson S, Sherrington R, Gurling H et al. Molecular genetic evidence of heterogeneity in manic-depression. *Nature* 1987; 325: 805–6.

(97) Detera-Wadleigh SD, Berrettini W, Goldin LR et al. Close linkage of c-Harvey-ras 1 and insulin gene to affective disorder is ruled out in three North American pedigrees. *Nature* 1987; 325: 806–8.

(98) Gill M, McKeon P, Humphries P. Linkage analysis of manic depression in an Irish family using H-ras 1 and INS DNA markers. *J Med Genet* 1988; 25: 634–7.

(99) Kelsoe JR, Ginns EI, Rgeland J et al. Re-evaluation of the linkage relationship between chromosome 11p loci and the gene for bipolar affective disorder in the Old Order Amish. *Nature* 1989; 342: 238–42.

(100) Tiwari J, Terasaki PI. *HLA and disease associations*. Berlin: Springer,1985.

(101) Mourant AE, Kopec AC, Domaniewska-Sobezak K. *Blood groups and diseases*. Oxford: Oxford University Press, 1978.

(102) Cooper DN, Clayton JF. DNA polymorphism and the study of disease associations. *Hum Genet* 1988; 78: 299–312.

(103) Sherrington R, Dixon P, Melmer G et al. Linkage disequilibrium between two highly polymorphic microsatellite sequences. *Am J Hum Genet* 1992; 49: 966–71.

(104) Ferns GA, Stocks J, Galton DJ. C-III DNA restriction fragment length polymorphism and myocardial infarction. *Lancet* 1986; i: 94.

(105) Sobell JL, Heston LL, Sommer SS. Delineation of genetic predisposition to multifactorial disease: a general approach on the threshold of feasibility. *Genomics* 1992; 12: 1–6.

(106) Vinogradov S, Gottesman II, Moises H et al. Negative association between schizophrenia and rheumatoid arthritis. *Schiz Bull* 1991; 17: 669–78.

(107) McGuffin P, Sturt P. Genetic markers in schizophrenia. *Hum Hered* 1986; 36: 65–88.

(108) Sanders A. Hamilton J, Fann W et al. Association of genetic variation at the porphobilinogen deaminase gene with schizophrenia. *Am J Hum Genet* 1991; 49: A2011.

(109) Owen M, Mant R, Parfitt E et al. A study of association between RFLPs at the porphobilinogen deaminase gene and schizophrenia. *Hum Genet*; in press.

(110) Nimgaonker VL, Washington SS, Ganguli R et al. An association study of schizophrenia and the porphobilinogen deaminase gene alleles. *Schizophrenia Res* 1992; 6: 90–1.

M Gill and C Walsh

(111) Todd RD, O'Malley K. Population frequencies of tyrosine hydroxylase restriction fragment length polymorphisms in bipolar affective disorder. *Biol Psych* 1989; 25: 626–30.

(112) Leboyer M, Malafosse A, Boularand S et al. Tyrosine hydroxylase polymorphisms associated with manic-depressive illness. *Lancet* 1990; 335: 1219.

(113) Korner J, Fritze J, Propping P. RFLP alleles at the tyrosine hydroxylase locus: no association found to affective disorders. *Psych Res* 1990; 32: 275–80.

(114) Gill M, Castle D, Hunt N et al. Tyrosine hydroxylase polymorphisms and bipolar affective disorder. *J Psych Res* 1991; 25: 177–84.

(115) Woolf B. On estimating the relation between blood groups and disease. *Ann Hum Genet* 1955; 19: 251–3.

Alzheimer's disease and the β-amyloid precursor protein

J HARDY

Introduction

The pathology of AD is complex: there are extracellular neuritic plaques, largely consisting of deposits of a peptide β-amyloid[1,2], intracellular neurofibrillary tangles largely consisting of overphosphorylated tau[3] and cell loss[4]. Pathological investigations have not allowed this complex pathology to be ordered ie it has not been possible to determine whether one aspect of the pathology comes first and causes the others, or whether they are independent sequelae of another primary event. Studies on Down's syndrome have, however, suggested that β-amyloid deposition is an early event in the process[5].

Genetics of AD

Occasionally, early onset AD segregates as an autosomal dominant disorder[6]. In one such family, we used molecular genetic techniques to identify a point mutation at codon 717, causing a valine to isoleucine change in APP[7]. This mutation has subsequently been detected in several other families with early onset AD, but not in the general population, sporadic cases of AD or late onset cases of AD whether familial or sporadic[7-10]. Thus this mutation is a rare cause of AD[7,11]. Subsequently, two other mutations at codon 717 have been described in single families: the first, changing valine to phenylalanine[12], the second, changing valine to glycine[13]. It is not yet clear whether mutations at other sites in the APP gene also lead to AD: however, these results clearly demonstrate that hereditary, early onset AD is allelically heterogeneous[14].

However, genetic linkage analysis clearly shows that there are many families, probably the majority, in which the APP gene does not segregate with early onset AD[15-18]. This contention is supported by the observation that

All correspondence to: Dr J Hardy, Alzheimer's Disease Research Group, Department of Biochemistry, St Mary's Hospital Medical School, London W2 1PG, UK.

the majority of families with early onset AD do not appear to have mutations in this gene[19,20]. Thus early onset, familial, AD also shows locus heterogeneity[17,18,21]. Genetic analysis has not yet allowed the location of the non-APP locus to be determined: indeed, there may be more than one other locus.

APP has several isoforms generated by alternative splicing of a 19 exon gene (exons 1–13, 13a, 14–18)[22]. The predominant transcripts are APP695 (exons 1–6, 9–18, not 13a), APP751 (exons 1–7, 9–18, not 13a) and APP770 (exons 1–18, not 13a). All of these encoded are multidomain proteins with a single transmembrane domain[23]. They differ in that APP751 and APP770 contain exon 7, which encodes a serine protease inhibitor domain[24–26]. APP695 is the predominant form in neuronal tissue: APP751, the predominant form elsewhere. β-amyloid is derived from that part of the protein encoded by parts of exons 16 and 17[22]. The β-amyloid section of the molecule is part within the membrane and part poking out into the extracellular space[23] (see Fig. 1). β-amyloid itself cannot be generated by alternative splicing and appears to be an abnormal proteolytic breakdown product[27]. The neural functions of APP are not known, but it is believed to be involved in synaptic contact[28] and as a growth regulating factor[29,30]. β-amyloid is believed to be solely a pathological byproduct of APP metabolism. So far, two metabolic pathways have been defined for the APP molecule. The first, 'secretase' pathway, apparently occurs at the cell membrane and involves cleavage at codon 687 (lysine) of APP (APP770 transcript): this cleavage is in the middle of the β-amyloid section of the molecule (codons 672–714) and precludes amyloidogenesis[31,32]. The second is in the β-amyloid fraction of the molecule leaving the β-amyloid containing stub within the membrane[33,34]. The precise site of this cleavage is not known but a likely site is at codon 670 (lysine).

The first pathogenic mutation described in APP was in a variant of CA: hereditary cerebral haemorrhage with angiopathy-Dutch type (HCHWA-D). This disease is characterized by massive β-amyloid depositions in cerebral vessels and death from strokes, typically in the fifth decade[35]. The disease is caused by a mutation changing glutamate to glutamine at codon 693 of the APP gene, in the middle of the β-amyloid sequence[36,37] (see Fig. 1). While the predominant feature of this disease is undoubtedly the vessel damage and there is little neuritic damage, it does seem as if there is a dementing process which occurs after, but independent of, this vessel damage[38].

Three different mutations, all causing AD have now been found at codon 717 of the APP gene, changing the native valine to isoleucine[7–10], phenylalanine[12] and glycine[13] (see Fig. 1). It seems likely that these APP mutations account for most, if not all, the evidence showing a chromosome 21 linkage for this disorder[39]. The controversy of this linkage[40,41] qv [17,42] being a result of the nonallelic genetic heterogeneity of the disorder[21]. All 33 of the APP717 mutations give rise to 'typical' AD with little CA[43,44]. This remark-

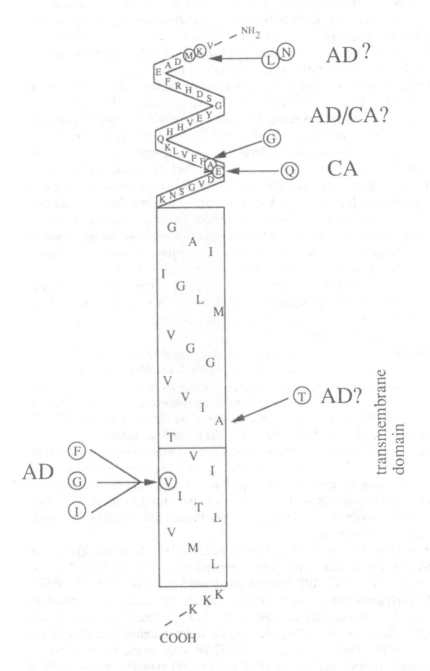

Fig. 1. Diagrammatic representation of the β-amyloid precursor protein (APP).

able clustering of mutations causing AD at a single codon led me, at least, to believe that these were likely to be the only mutations causing AD. However, a recent series of experiments to be published by several groups makes this conclusion less likely, and suggests that the genotype/phenotype correlations for APP mutations is likely to be complex and interesting.

Hendriks and colleagues report a mutation transposing alanine for glycine at codon 692. This mutation is adjacent to that causing HCHWA-D, and on this basis, it is perhaps not surprising that some individuals with the mutation develop a disease very similar to HCHWA-D. More surprising, however, is the fact that some individuals develop neuritic plaques and a dementing disorder which may be full blown AD (the lack of detailed, postmortem neuropathology makes a definitive diagnosis, for which neurofibrillary tangles are required, difficult). While it is formally possible that there are two diseases segregating within the family (the occurrence of a demented person without a mutation could be adduced to support this conclusion), it would seem most parsimonious to assume that the single demented case without the mutation is a case of 'sporadic' dementia. Thus the mutation APP692Ala→Gly seems to cause a 'flickering' phenotype, with two distinct clinical courses and (presumably) pathological outcomes. Detailed neuropathology on cases with this mutation will be required before definitive statements can be made.

Mullan, Lannfelt and their colleagues have identified two families in which a double mutation at the same site (APP670/671 Lys/Met→Asn/Leu) segregates with NINCDS-probable AD. The positions of these mutations are interesting because they are close to, or at the endosomal/lysosomal cleavage site for, APP[33,34] at the N-terminal of β-amyloid. In contrast, the APP717 mutations are close to the C-terminal of the β-amyloid moiety.

Can these mutations be put together in a rational genotype→phenotype series? The simple answer is 'not yet'. As in prion disease, where prion mutations have unexpected phenotypes, so it would seem in APP diseases. However, it is probably worthwhile trying to put forward a tentative scheme of genotype→phenotype relationships, even though this is likely to be wrong in many of its elements.

It is clear that APP717 mutations cause AD[45]. It seems likely that APP670/671 also causes AD. These mutations are at either end of the β-amyloid section of the APP molecules and could be hypothesized to stabilize APP derivatives containing β-amyloid slightly by inhibition of proteases which digest preamyloid deposits in the brain parenchyma. In contrast, APP693Glu→Gln causes CA, and may do so by marginal inhibition of the 'secretase'[31,32]. On this scheme, APP692Ala→Gly would be predicted to marginally inhibit both the 'secretase' and the endosomal/lysosomal pathway to a similar extent, and the resultant variable phenotype would be predicted to reflect the relative inhibition in the two pathways.

Clearly much more work needs to be done before any certainty can be assigned to genotype/phenotype interaction in APP disease. Most sequencing and screening effort has been directed at exon 17 (amino acids 688–730 of APP) in both CA and AD. Clearly, much more needs to be done to screen other exons of the gene for variability in psychiatric disorders and, most importantly, in normal controls so that the variability in APP sequence can be defined as well as its role in disease. We have just completed a screen of the entire open reading frame of the APP gene in 12 families with early onset familial AD without finding novel mutations[46]. The papers reviewed here indicate that this arduous task needs to be continued.

References

(1) Masters CL, Simms G, Weinman NA et al. Amyloid plaque core protein in Alzheimer disease and Down syndrome. *Proc Nat Acad Sci USA* 1985; 82: 4245–9.

(2) Glenner GG, Wong CW. Alzheimer's disease: initial report of the purification and characterization of a novel cerebrovascular amyloid protein. *Biochem Biophys Res Commun* 1984; 120: 885–90.

(3) Lee VM, Balin BJ, Otvos LJ et al. A68: a major subunit of paired helical filaments and derivatized forms of normal Tau. *Science* 1991; 251: 675–8.

(4) Mann DM, Yates PO, Marcyniuk B et al. Loss of neurones from cortical and subcortical areas in Down's syndrome patients at middle age. Quantitative comparisons with younger Down's patients and patients with Alzheimer's disease. *J Neurol Sci* 1987; 80: 79–89.

(5) Mann DM, Esiri MM. The pattern of acquisition of plaques and tangles in the brains of patients under 50 years of age with Down's syndrome. *J Neurol Sci* 1989; 89: 169–79.

(6) St George Hyslop PH, Myers RH, Haines JL et al. Familial Alzheimer's disease: progress and problems. *Neurobiol Aging* 1989; 10: 417–27.

(7) Goate A, Chartier-Harlin MC, Mullan M et al. Segregation of a missense mutation in the amyloid precursor protein gene with familial Alzheimer's disease. *Nature* 1991; 349: 704–6.

(8) Naruse S, Igarashi S, Kobayashi H et al. Mis-sense mutation Val→Ile in exon 17 of amyloid precursor protein gene in Japanese familial Alzheimer's disease. *Lancet* 1991; 337: 978–9.

(9) Yoshioka K, Miki T, Katsuya T et al. The [717]Val→Ile substitution in amyloid precursor protein is associated with familial Alzheimer's disease regardless of ethnic groups. *Biochem Biophys Res Commun* 1991; 178: 1141–6.

(10) Hardy J, Mullan M, Chartier-Harlin MC et al. Molecular classification of Alzheimer's disease. *Lancet* 1991; 337: 1342–3.

(11) van Duijn CM, Hendriks L, Cruts M et al. Amyloid precursor protein gene mutation in early-onset Alzheimer's disease. *Lancet* 1991; 337: 978.

(12) Murrell J, Farlow M, Ghetti B et al. A mutation in the amyloid precursor protein associated with hereditary Alzheimer's disease. *Science* 1991; 254: 97–9.

(13) Chartier-Harlin MC, Crawford F, Houlden H et al. Early onset Alzheimer's

disease caused by mutations at codon 717 of the β-amyloid precursor protein gene. *Nature* 1991; 353: 844–6.

(14) van Duijn CM, Van Broeckhoven C, Hardy JA et al. Evidence for allelic heterogeneity in familial early onset Alzheimer's disease. *Br J Psych* 1991; 158: 471–4.

(15) Tanzi RE, St George Hyslop PH, Haines JL et al. The genetic defect in familial Alzheimer's disease is not tightly linked to the amyloid β-protein gene. *Nature* 1987; 329: 156–7.

(16) Van Broeckhoven C, Genthe AM, Vandenberghe A et al. Failure of familial Alzheimer's disease to segregate with the A4 amyloid gene in several European families. *Nature* 1987; 329: 153–5.

(17) Schellenberg GD, Bird TD, Wijsman EM et al. Absence of linkage of chromosome 21q21 markers to familial Alzheimer's disease. *Science* 1988; 241: 1507–10.

(18) Schellenberg GD, Pericak Vance MA, Wijsman EM et al. Linkage analysis of familial Alzheimer disease, using chromosome 21 markers. *Am J Hum Genet* 1991; 48: 563–83.

(19) Chartier-Harlin MC, Crawford F, Hamandi K et al. Screening for the β-amyloid precursor protein mutation (APP:Val→Ile) in extended pedigrees with early onset Alzheimer's disease. *Neurosci Lett* 1991; 129: 134–5.

(20) Crawford F, Hardy J, Mullan M et al. Sequencing of exons 16 and 17 of the β-amyloid precursor protein gene in families with early onset Alzheimer's disease fails to reveal mutations in the β-amyloid sequence. *Neurosci Lett* 1991; 133: 1–2.

(21) St George Hyslop PH, Haines JL, Farrer LA et al. Genetic linkage studies suggest that Alzheimer's disease is not a single homogeneous disorder. FAD Collaborative Study Group. *Nature* 1990; 347: 194–7.

(22) Yoshikai S, Sasaki H, Dohura K et al. Genomic organization of the human amyloid beta-protein precursor gene. *Gene* 1990; 87: 257–63.

(23) Kang J, Lemaire HG, Unterbeck A et al. The precursor of Alzheimer's disease amyloid A4 protein resembles a cell-surface receptor. *Nature* 1987; 325: 733–6.

(24) Ponte P, Gonzalez-De Whitt P, Schilling J et al. A new A4 amyloid mRNA contains a domain homologous to serine protease inhibitors. *Nature* 1988; 331: 525–7.

(25) Kitaguchi N, Takahashi Y, Tokushima Y et al. Novel precursor of Alzheimer's disease amyloid protein shows protease inhibitory activity. *Nature* 1988; 331: 530–2.

(26) Tanzi RE, McClatchey AI, Lamberti ED et al. Protease inhibitor domain encoded by an amyloid precursor mRNA associated with Alzheimer's disease. *Nature* 1988; 331: 528–30.

(27) Lemaire HG, Salbaum JM, Multhaup G et al. The PreA4(695) precursor protein of Alzheimer's disease A4 amyloid is encoded by 16 exons. *Nucl Acids Res* 1989; 17: 517–22.

(28) Schubert W, Prior R, Weidemann A et al. Localization of Alzheimer β/A4 amyloid precursor protein at central and peripheral synaptic sites. *Brain Res* 1991; 563: 184–94.

(29) Oltersdorf T, Fritz LC, Schenk DB et al. The secreted form of the Alzheimer's

amyloid precursor protein with the Kunitz domain is protease nexin-II. *Nature* 1989; 341: 144–7.

(30) Van Nostrand WE, Farrow JS, Wagner SL et al. The predominant form of the amyloid β-protein precursor in human brain is protease nexin 2. *Proc Nat Acad Sci USA* 1991; 88: 10302–6.

(31) Esch FS, Keim PS, Beattie EC et al. Cleavage of amyloid beta peptide during constitutive processing of its precursor. *Science* 1990; 248: 1122–4.

(32) Anderson JP, Esch FS, Keim PS et al. Exact cleavage site of Alzheimer amyloid precursor in neuronal PC-12 cells. *Neurosci Lett* 1991; 128: 126–8.

(33) Estus S, Golde TE, Kunishita T et al. Potentially amyloidogenic, carboxyl terminal derivatives of the amyloid protein precursor. *Science* 1992; 255: 726–8.

(34) Golde TE, Estus S, Younkin LH et al. Processing of the amyloid protein precursor to potentially amyloidogenic fragments. *Science* 1992; 255: 728–30.

(35) van Duinen SG, Castano EM, Prelli F et al. Hereditary cerebral hemorrhage with amyloidosis in patients of Dutch origin is related to Alzheimer disease. *Proc Nat Acad Sci USA* 1987; 84: 5991–4.

(36) Levy E, Carman MD, Fernandez Madrid IJ et al. Mutation of the Alzheimer's disease amyloid gene in hereditary cerebral hemorrhage, Dutch type. *Science* 1990; 248: 1124–6.

(37) Van Broeckhoven C, Haan J, Bakker E et al. Amyloid beta protein precursor gene and hereditary cerebral hemorrhage with amyloidosis (Dutch). *Science* 1990; 248: 1120–2.

(38) Haan J, Roos RA, Algra PR et al. Hereditary cerebral haemorrhage with amyloidosis–Dutch type. Magnetic resonance imaging findings in 7 cases. *Brain* 1990; 113: 1251–67.

(39) Hardy J, Chartier-Harlin MC, Mullan M. Alzheimer disease: the new agenda. *Am J Hum Genet* 1992; 50: 648–51.

(40) St George Hyslop PH, Tanzi RE, Polinsky RJ et al. The genetic defect causing familial Alzheimer's disease maps on chromosome 21. *Science* 1987; 235: 885–90.

(41) Goate AM, Haynes AR, Owen MJ et al. Predisposing locus for Alzheimer's disease on chromosome 21. *Lancet* 1989; 1: 352–5.

(42) Pericak-Vance MA, Yamaoka LH, Haynes CS et al. Genetic linkage studies in familial Alzheimer's disease. *Exp Neurol* 1988; 102: 271–9.

(43) Mann DMA, Jones D, Snowden JS et al. Pathological changes in the brain of a patient with familial Alzheimer's disease having a missense mutation at codon 717 in the amyloid precursor protein gene. *Neurosci Lett* 1992; 137: 225–8.

(44) Lantos PL, Luthert PJ, Hanger D et al. Familial Alzheimer's disease with the amyloid precursor protein position 717 mutation and sporadic Alzheimer's disease have the same cytoskeletal pathology. *Neurosci Lett* 1992; 137: 221–4.

(45) Hardy JA, Higgins GA. Alzheimer's disease: the amyloid cascade hypothesis. *Science* 1992; 286: 184–5.

(46) Fidani L, Rooke K, Chartier-Harlin MC et al. Screening for mutations in the open reading frame and promoter of the β-amyloid precursor protein gene in familial Alzheimer's disease: identification of a further family with APP717 Val→Ile. *Hum Mol Genet* 1992; in press.

The biochemistry of tau proteins in Alzheimer's disease

J-M GALLO

Introduction

Alzheimer's disease is a disorder of old age characterized by progressive neuronal cell death in selective areas of the brain, mainly the hippocampus and the cerebral cortex, causing failure of memory and cognitive functions and dementia.

Two major neuropathological lesions are recognized in Alzheimer's disease brain: extracellular amyloid plaques and neurofibrillary tangles in the cell bodies of degenerating neurones. Amyloid plaques are made of the β/A4 peptide which is derived from the proteolytic processing of a larger precursor, the amyloid precursor protein or APP.

Neurofibrillary tangles are aggregates of paired helical filaments that are pairs of filaments of an approximate diameter of 10 nm helically twisted about each other with a half periodicity of 80 nm. Paired helical filaments are also found in dystrophic neurites associated with plaques and neuropil threads.

The filamentous structure of paired helical filaments together with the disruption of the cytoskeleton of vulnerable neurones, as observed on biopsy material[1,2], led to the early assumption that paired helical filaments were derived from the neuronal cytoskeleton. Immunological and biochemical studies have shown that it was indeed the case and the biochemical composition of paired helical filaments has been reviewed in an earlier chapter of this series[3]. Recent developments in the molecular biology of Alzheimer's disease have made clear that the main component of paired helical filaments, tau proteins, have, in Alzheimer's disease brain, properties that distinguish them from their counterpart in normal brain.

It is now clear from genetic studies[4,5] that the amyloid precursor protein (APP) is central to the pathological process of Alzheimer's disease. A better understanding of the mechanisms of cytoskeletal pathology in Alzheimer's

All correspondence to: Dr J-M Gallo, Department of Neurology, Institute of Psychiatry and King's College School of Medicine and Dentistry, De Crespigny Park, London SE5 8AF, UK.

Cambridge Medical Reviews: Neurobiology and Psychiatry Volume 2
© Cambridge University Press

disease and how they relate to APP metabolism would give a complete picture of the pathogenesis of Alzheimer's disease as well as provide several potential targets for drug therapy. The aim of this review is to give an overview of today's understanding of the biochemistry of tau in paired helical filaments in the light of recent discoveries in this field.

Evidence for tau as the main component of paired helical filaments
The main breakthrough in the biochemistry of paired helical filaments came from the discovery that their main component was the microtubule associated protein, tau. Tau proteins are members of the family of proteins that copurify with microtubules, the so-called microtubule associated proteins or MAPs, and promote tubulin polymerization. Tau proteins have a molecular mass ranging from 47 kD to 63 kD, they are specifically neuronal and mainly found in axons.

Tau has been found to be a main component of paired helical filaments by both immunochemical and biochemical methods. Antibodies to tau stain neurofibrillary tangles in tissue sections from Alzheimer's disease brain[6-9] and antibodies raised against PHF-enriched fractions recognize tau in microtubule preparations from mouse and human fetal brain[7,9].

Until recently, the insolubility of paired helical filaments in SDS had precluded any direct biochemical analysis of their protein composition. The first attempt to do so has been by Wischik and colleagues[10] who exploited the SDS insolubility of neurofibrillary tangles to obtain them in a reasonably pure form, as confirmed by electron microscopy. Pronase treatment of such purified paired helical filaments released several peptides. The sequence of one of these peptides was used to design oligonucleotide probes to clone a cDNA coding for the protein it was derived from[11]. The sequence of this cDNA was found to have a high degree of homology with the then recently published sequence of mouse tau[12]. Kondo and colleagues[13] also isolated and sequenced peptides from paired helical filaments and from human tau and found that paired helical filaments peptides were derived from tau.

Taking advantage of the existence of a non-aggregated population of paired helical filaments soluble in SDS, methods of purification of SDS-soluble paired helical filaments have been devised providing preparations that could readily be analyzed by SDS-PAGE and Western blotting[14-16]. This has revealed that the main component of paired helical filaments was resolved as a group of polypeptides of an apparent molecular weight of 57–68 kD, distinct, in term of apparent molecular weight from normal brain tau (47–63 kD), but reacting with all antibodies to tau used. In these preparations, tau appears as three bands with an overall higher electrophoretic mobility than normal brain tau.

Flament and colleagues also observed that antibodies to tau stained two bands of 64 and 69 kD in total homogenates from Alzheimer's disease brain that were absent from control brains[17-19].

The form(s) of tau present in paired helical filaments received different names, including A68, PHF-tau, τmb $_{PHF}$, tau 64 and tau 69. Although still debated by some authors, the current evidence is that these different names represent the same biochemical entity that will be referred to as PHF-tau in this review.

PHF-tau is composed of all tau isoforms

Six isoforms of tau are expressed in the human central nervous system; they are generated by alternative RNA splicing and contain either three or four copies of a tandemly repeated homologous 31 amino-acid sequence in their C-terminal half[20-22]. In addition, they contain none, 1 or 2 N-terminal 29 amino acid inserts[21] (Fig. 1). The C-terminal repeated motifs are microtubule binding sites[23]. The whole complement of tau isoforms is expressed in adult brain; the shortest isoform, with three C-terminal motifs and no N-terminal motif (352 amino acid isoform), is the only one expressed in fetal brain[21].

Immunocytochemical mapping using panels of monoclonal or antipeptide antibodies spanning the tau molecule has demonstrated that the whole of the tau molecule was incorporated in paired helical filaments[24,25].

Peptides isolated from paired helical filament preparations contain sequences overlapping domains C1 and C3 of tau as well as sequences included in the C2 domain[10,13,26] (see Fig. 1), therefore 3 and 4-repeat forms of tau are present in paired helical filaments.

An immunochemical analysis of PHF-tau using antibodies against peptides specific for the N-terminal inserts of tau led to the conclusion that PHF-tau was composed of the whole complement of tau isoforms[16,27]. This was further confirmed by the electrophoretic analysis of dephosphorylated PHF-tau that ran as six bands in SDS-PAGE, comigrating with recombinant isoforms of tau produced in bacteria[16].

State of phosphorylation of PHF-tau

Although normally phosphorylated in brain, the main feature distinguishing PHF-tau from tau is its state of phosphorylation. The evidence for this are both biochemical and immunochemical.

The stoichiometry of phosphorylation of PHF-tau has been estimated to be 11 phosphates/molecule as compared to 4 phosphates/molecule for normal tau[28]. This indicates that PHF-tau is an hyperphosphorylated form of tau.

As mentioned earlier, PHF-tau has a reduced electrophoretic mobility in gels as compared to normal tau. Flament and colleagues observed that the 2 tau immunoreactive bands of 64 and 69 kD specifically found in homogenates from Alzheimer's disease brain disappeared after treatment with alkaline phosphatase[17-19]. Similarly, treatment of PHF-tau preparations with alkaline

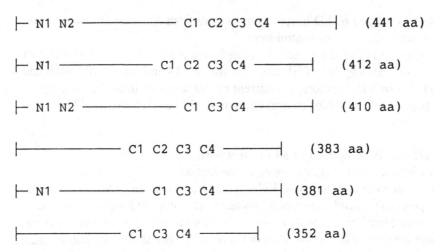

Fig. 1. Schematic representation of the six tau isoforms expressed in the human central nervous system.

phosphatase results in an increased mobility of tau[14,15]. More precisely, complete dephosphorylation of PHF-tau transforms the characteristic 3-band pattern of PHF-tau into a 6-band pattern, each band aligning with one of recombinant tau isoforms[16]. Therefore the abnormal electrophoretic migration of PHF-tau is the result of a specific type of tau phosphorylation occurring in Alzheimer's disease; this type of phosphorylation induces an electrophoretic shift of all tau isoforms.

A reduced electrophoretic mobility of tau following phosphorylation by some kinases can be obtained in vitro by several kinases including Ca^{2+}/calmodulin dependent kinase[15,29] and cAMP-dependent protein kinase[30,31] and a number of proline-directed kinases (see below). An explanation for the retardation in gels is provided by the major change in tau structure observed following phosphorylation. The tau molecule has a rod-like shape[32] and electron microscopy observations of paracrystals of tau have revealed that the tau molecule stretches upon phosphorylation by Ca^{2+}/calmodulin dependent kinase[33].

The other line of evidence for an abnormal phosphorylation of tau in Alzheimer's disease comes from the analysis of the properties of a number of monoclonal antibodies binding to tau in a phosphorylation-dependent manner. The first of these antibodies is the monoclonal antibody, tau 1, produced against bovine brain tau[34], that stains neurofibrillary tangles only if the sections have been treated with alkaline phosphatase prior to immunostaining[35]. Similarly, the reactivity of tau 1 on Western blots of brain extract from AD is greatly enhanced by treatment of nitrocellulose sheets with alkaline phosphatase prior to antibody staining[35]. Conversely, the monoclonal

Table 1. *Marker antibodies of the phosphorylayion state of PHF-tau. Amino acid residues are identified by their position on the longest tau isoform (441 amino acids)*

Antibody	Tau	PHF-tau	Serine residue(s) involved
Tau 1	+	−	199 and/or 202
AT8	−	+	199 and/or 202
SMI33	+	−	235
Anti-T3	+	−	396
Anti-T3P	−	+	396
SMI31	−	+	396 and 404
SMI34	−	+	

antibody AT8[36], produced against paired helical filaments and the antiserum anti-T3P[37], elicited against a chemically phosphorylated peptide, exclusively bind to PHF-tau and the binding is abolished by dephosphorylation. The properties of these antibodies and of a few others are summarized in Table 1.

Phosphorylation sites of PHF-tau
The knowledge of the position of aberrantly phosphorylated sites in PHF-tau is important to investigate further the metabolic processes involved in tau hyperphosphorylation in Alzheimer's disease. Several of these aberrantly phosphorylated sites have now been localized. They will be identified here by their position in the longest isoform of tau, ie the 441 amino acid isoform.

Polyclonal antibodies have been produced against a synthetic peptide corresponding to residues 389 to 402 of tau (anti-T3) and against the same peptide phosphorylated chemically (anti-T3P)[37]. Anti-T3P does not recognize the native peptide in which the only residue that can undergo phosphorylation is Ser[396]. Since anti-T3P binds to PHF-tau and not to normal tau (see above), Ser[396] is likely to be phosphorylated in PHF-tau.

The epitope for tau 1 was shown to be comprised between residues Pro[189] and Gly[207] of tau[24]. Sequencing of peptides phosphorylated by a brain kinase showed that the monoclonal antibody AT8, specific for PHF-tau, recognized the phosphorylated version of the same epitope as tau 1 and that phosphorylation at Ser[199] and/or Ser[202] was required for AT8 binding[36].

Another site would be between residues 119 and 131[25] as well as one close to the N-terminus of tau[38].

Neurofibrillary tangles have long been known to share antigenic

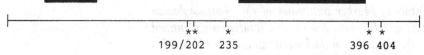

Fig. 2. Position of the putative phosphorylation sites of PHF-tau on the longest isoform of tau (441 amino acids). Top bars indicate the position of the N-terminal insert domains and the microtubule-binding domains.

determinants with the middle and heavy chain of neurofilaments, NF-M and NF-H[39-41]. There is a number of monoclonal antibodies cross-reacting with NF-M/NF-H and neurofibrillary tangles and most of them recognize multiphosphorylation domains which contain repeated Lys–Ser–Pro[41,42]. Tau possesses two such sequences: Lys–Ser[235]–Pro and Lys–Ser[396]–Pro. The antibodies SMI31, SMI33 and SMI34 all bind to the multiphosphorylation domain of neurofilaments and their reactivity is dependent upon the phosphorylation state of this domain[40,43]. SMI33 also binds to normal tau but not to PHF-tau, but SMI33 recognizes dephosphorylated PHF-tau[44]. Conversely, SMI31 and SMI34 recognize PHF-tau and not normal tau; the binding of SMI31 and SMI34 on PHF-tau is abolished by dephosphorylation[44]. Recombinant tau phosphorylated by a kinase isolated from brain (see below) displays the same pattern of immunoreactivity and was used to identify the epitopes for SMI31 and SMI33. The binding of SMI31 to PHF-tau requires phosphorylation at both Ser[396] and Ser[404], and phosphorylation at Ser[235] abolishes the binding of SMI33 to tau. Thus, in addition to Ser[199] and/or Ser[202] and Ser[396], PHF-tau is likely to be phosphorylated at Ser[235] and Ser[404].

The position of all the putative phosphorylation sites of PHF-tau known to date are summarized in Fig. 2. According to the stoichiometry of phosphorylation of PHF-tau (11 phosphates/molecule in PHF tau vs 4 phosphates/molecules in normal tau[28]) several sites remain to be identified.

Putative kinases involved in the generation of PHF-tau
Identifying the kinases responsible for the transformation of tau into PHF-tau is important to understand the mechanisms of PHF formation and would eventually lead to the discovery of putative targets for drug therapy. In terms of phosphorylation, PHF-tau is characterized by a reduced electrophoretic mobility and by phosphorylation at residues Ser[199]/Ser[202] and Ser[396]. The site-specific phosphorylation can be easily probed by the reactivity of antibodies like tau 1/AT8 and anti-T3P, respectively. Putative Alzheimer's kinase(s) can therefore be assayed by reconstituting these properties in vitro on dephosphorylated brain tau or on bacterially synthesized recombinant tau. This approach has been used for known kinases or kinases activities purified from mammalian brain.

It is noteworthy that all the aberrantly phosphorylated sites in PHF-tau identified to date are serine residues followed by a proline residue. Such sites are phosphorylated by a class of serine/threonine kinases, the so-called proline directed kinases. Among proline directed kinases are the cell cycle regulated kinase p34^{cdc2} kinase and the mitogen activated protein kinases (MAP kinases) that are activated by tyrosine phosphorylation in response to growth factors.

A MAP kinase from *Xenopus* oocytes has been used to phosphorylate recombinant tau, it induces an electrophoretic shift as well as phosphorylation at Ser[199]/Ser[202] and at several other sites including the site(s) recognized by the monoclonal antibody SMI31; consequently, Ser[396] and Ser[404] are likely to be phosphorylated by the MAP kinase from *Xenopus* oocytes.

By contrast, complexes of p34^{cdc2} kinase and either cyclin A or cyclin B, although they phosphorylate tau, fail to induce an electrophoretic shift or produce any immunoreactivity characteristic of PHF-tau[45].

Recombinant tau can also be phosphorylated in vitro by other kinases, inducing an electrophoretic shift, like Ca^{2+}/calmodulin dependent kinase[29] and cAMP-dependent protein kinase[30,31], or not, like protein kinase C[29]; however, none of them has been reported to induce phosphorylation at sites characteristic of PHF-tau.

Kinase activities inducing PHF-tau-like properties on tau have also been purified from brain tissue. Mandelkow and colleagues[36,45] purified from porcine brain a 42 kD kinase activity possessing properties of MAP kinases, ie molecular mass of 40–45 kD, activation by tyrosine phosphorylation, reaction with an antibody to a conserved epitope of MAP kinases. This kinase incorporates 14 to 16 phosphates in tau and induces electrophoretic and antigenic properties characteristic of PHF-tau. A similar MAP kinase activity has been also found in extracts from postmortem brain from Alzheimer's disease patients[45]. Roder and Ingram[46] have isolated from bovine brain two kinases, PK36 and PK40, 36 kD and 40 kD, respectively, inducing an electrophoretic shift of tau as well as the reactivity of the monoclonal antibody SMI34. Ishiguro and colleagues[47,48] reported the presence in bovine brain of a kinase activity stimulated by tubulin and phosphorylating tau and shifting it on gels as well as inducing a PHF-epitope. These authors subsequently purified this activity as a 45 kD protein referred to as TPKI[49]. TPKI decreases tau 1 immunoreactivity and phosphorylates a tau peptide containing Ser/Thr-Pro motifs and was therefore considered to be a proline directed kinase.

In situ properties of PHF-tau: the monoclonal antibody Alz 50
The monoclonal antibody, Alz 50, has been produced by Davies and colleagues after immunization of mice with Alzheimer's disease brain homogenates[50]. Alz 50 does recognize all tau isoforms as well as PHF-tau on Western blots and therefore appears to be a *bona fide* antitau antibody[51,52].

However, Alz 50 departs from other anti-tau antibodies by its immuno-histochemical properties. Applied to sections of Alzheimer's disease brain, Alz 50 stains neurofibrillary tangles as well as the cytoplasm of neurones that do not display any neurofibrillary pathology[50,53]. Alz 50 does not show any reactivity with brain sections from normal individuals.

This suggests that the Alz 50 epitope becomes accessible to the antibody by a conformational change of tau preceding its accumulation in paired helical filaments and that Alz 50 stains vulnerable neurones before they bear neuro-fibrillary tangles and can be used as a marker of early stages of neurofibrillary degeneration.

Several laboratories have attempted to localize the Alz 50 epitope on tau and came to different conclusions.

By analysing Alz 50 reactivity to proteolytic fragments of human tau, Ksiezak-Reding and colleagues[54] concluded that the Alz 50 epitope was located within 3–4 kD of the N-terminus of tau. By using a similar approach, Uéda and colleagues[55] found that the Alz 50 epitope was in the carboxy terminus of tau, within a 14 amino acid sequence next to the 31 amino acid repeat cluster. These authors further suggested that Alz 50 recognized a phosphorylated epitope sensitive to acid phosphatase. The idea that Alz 50 may recognize a phosphorylated epitope is supported by the properties of a kinase copurifying with paired helical filaments the inhibition of which abolishes Alz 50 reactivity on PHF-tau[56].

Although divergent, these results are in agreement with the early observation that Alz 50 does not bind to recombinant tau[24]. However, Goedert and colleagues found that Alz 50 recognized all human recombinant tau isoforms expressed in bacteria[57]. By screening partial tau clones, these authors mapped the Alz 50 epitope between amino acids 2 to 10 of tau, a result confirmed in immunohistochemistry since the staining was abolished by absorption with the corresponding peptide[57].

Is PHF-tau ubiquitinated?
The protein other than tau which is undoubtedly present in paired helical filaments is the 8 kD protein ubiquitin. Mori and colleagues[58] first identified ubiquitin as a component of neurofibrillary tangles by amino acid sequencing of peptides released from PHF fractions by protease treatment. This result was confirmed by using specific antibodies to ubiquitin in immuno-histochemistry on sections from Alzheimer's disease brain and paired helical filament preparations. As a matter of fact, ubiquitin is present in all inclusion bodies derived from the cytoskeleton that are characteristic of several diseases including most neurodegenerative diseases[59].

Antibodies to ubiquitin only label 50% of intracellular neurofibrillary tangles in situ, but this percentage reaches 95% in SDS-isolated paired helical filaments indicating that ubiquitin is either masked in situ in a subpopulation of neurofibrillary tangles or associated to an insoluble subpopulation of paired helical filaments[60].

The best known of ubiquitin's physiological functions is that it covalently binds to short-lived or abnormal proteins committed to rapid degradation by an ATP-dependent pathway. Since PHF-tau is, by some aspects, an abnormal form of tau, it is reasonable to assume that it may be ubiquitinated. The presence of ubiquitin in paired helical filaments may simply reflect the attempt of the cell to dispose of an abnormal protein. Nevertheless, ubiquitination of PHF-tau is still awaiting firm demonstration and this may be due to the known difficulty of detecting ubiquitinated proteins by conventional immunochemical methods. The monoclonal antibodies 3–39 and 5–25 raised against paired helical filaments and found to recognize sequences 50–65 and 64–76, of ubiquitin, respectively[61], react, on PHF preparations, with bands comigrating with bands stained by antibodies to tau, but they do not stain tau prepared from human or bovine brain[62]. Vincent and Davies[63] found that incubation of PHF-tau-containing fractions in the presence of ATP resulted in the loss of the Alz 50 epitope and that this process was inhibited by antibodies to ubiquitin. In addition, PHF-tau was immunoprecipitated by the same antibodies to ubiquitin. These authors concluded that PHF-tau might be a ubiquitin acceptor in Alzheimer's disease brain.

Although the cellular scavenger role for ubiquitin is an attractive one to explain its coaccumulation with tau in paired helical filaments, it should be noted that ubiquitin can be conjugated to proteins not committed to enhanced degradation like histones H2A and H2B, and has probably other roles in cellular function.

Tau hyperphosphorylation and cytoskeletal pathology

The two main features of cytoskeletal pathology in Alzheimer's disease are the disruption of microtubules in affected neurones and the accumulation of tau in paired helical filaments in an hyperphosphorylated state.

The primary event may be tau hyperphosphorylation, and phosphorylated tau would not bind to microtubules. Indeed, phosphorylation appears to regulate the binding of tau to microtubules since dephosphorylated tau is more potent at promoting microtubule assembly in vitro than native tau[64]. Furthermore there are some reports showing that PHF-tau is not capable of binding to microtubules[37,65].

The lack of binding of tau to microtubules would be in itself enough to disrupt axonal microtubules; indeed, experiments using antisense techniques have shown that tau was necessary for both differentiation and maintenance of axonal processes in cerebellar neurones in primary culture[66,67].

Alternatively, the Alzheimer-type phosphorylation of tau may be a normal feature of tau unbound to microtubules and microtubule depolymerization could be the primary event leaving tau free in the cytoplasm where it would become phosphorylated. This hypothesis is supported by the increased immunoreactivity for tau antibodies, including Alz 50, in cultured neurones treated with the microtubule-depolymerizing drug colchicine[68]. In both cases, tau would be free in the cytoplasm but would accumulate in paired helical filaments rather than being disposed of. However, other MAPs would also be released in the cytoplasm as the result of microtubule disruption but would not accumulate in paired helical filaments to the same extent as tau. This may be because phosphorylation protects tau from degradation. Indeed, phosphorylation of tau by cAMP-dependent protein kinase protects tau from degradation by calpains[30].

Amyloid deposition and cytoskeletal pathology

Recent genetic evidence[4,5] has demonstrated that mutations in the amyloid precursor protein from which the β/A4 peptide composing plaques is derived, can cause Alzheimer's disease. Brain tissue from a patient with a valine→isoleucine mutation at codon 717 of the APP gene displays the same cytoskeletal pathology as tissue from sporadic Alzheimer's disease[69], therefore demonstrating that the cytoskeletal pathology is a consequence of the abnormal properties of APP. Furthermore, PHF-tau isolated from this specimen is indistinguishable from PHF-tau produced in sporadic Alzheimer's disease[69]. Similarly, PHF-tau is found in brain tissue from patients with Down's syndrome[15,70] that develop an Alzheimer-type pathology presumably as a consequence of higher level of APP expression due to the extra copy of chromosome 21 on which the gene coding for APP is localized. Thus the transformation of tau into PHF-tau appears to be central to the cytoskeletal pathology of Alzheimer's disease.

How abnormal APP processing leads to cytoskeletal pathology in nerve cells is still unknown, however there is recent evidence that extracellular accumulation of the β/A4 peptide is capable of inducing tau alterations in several experimental systems.

SDS-isolated amyloid cores or a peptide corresponding to residues 1 to 40 of β/A4 have been introduced into the cerebral cortex or the hippocampus of rats by stereotaxic injection. These treatments caused focal degeneration of neurones near the site of injection as well as induced Alz 50 immunoreactivity[71,72]. Amyloid-like fibrils are formed in nonneuronal cells transfected with a vector expressing the C-terminal 104 amino acid fragment of APP spanning the cytoplasmic domain of APP and the β/A4 peptide[73]. Neve and colleagues had shown that pheochromocytoma cells (PC12) transfected with a similar vector degenerated when induced to differentiate by nerve growth factor[74]. Four months after transplantation of transfected PC12 cells into the brain of newborn mice, significant cortical atrophy was observed as well as Alz 50 immunoreactivity[75].

The β/A4 peptide is not toxic per se on cultured mouse cortical neurones, but enhances their vulnerability to excitotoxic damage[76]. Mattson and colleagues reported the same effect on cultured human cortical neurones[77] and showed that it was not specific to a particular subtype of glutamate receptor. β/A4 acts by elevating the rest level of intracellular calcium and by enhancing calcium entry resulting from glutamate receptor stimulation. A consequence of calcium entry, produced by either glutamate or ionophore treatment, is an increased immunoreactivity for tau antibodies, including Alz 50, that may be the consequence of microtubule disruption[68,77,78].

Conclusion
It is now clear that the abnormal phosphorylation of tau is central to the intracellular events downstream to amyloid deposition eventually leading to neuronal cell death. Deciphering the metabolic pathways involved is now well under way and the rapid progress in this field will hopefully provide in a not too distant future targets for drug therapy to counteract or slow down the pathological process of Alzheimer's disease.

References
(1) Flament-Durand J, Couck A-M. Spongiform alterations in brain biopsies of presenile dementia. *Acta Neuropathol* 1979; 46: 159–62.
(2) Gray EG, Paula-Barbosa M, Roher A. Alzheimer's disease: paired helical filaments and cytomembranes. *Neuropath Appl Neurobiol* 1987; 13: 91–110.
(3) Goedert M, Potier MC and Spillantini MG. Molecular neuropathology of Alzheimer's disease. In: Kerwin R ed. *Cambridge medical reviews: neurobiology and psychiatry* Volume 1, Cambridge: Cambridge University Press, 1991: 95–118.
(4) Goate A, Chartier-Harlin MC, Mullan M et al. Segregation of a missense mutation in the amyloid precursor protein gene with familial Alzheimer's disease. *Nature* 1991; 349: 704–6.
(5) Chartier-Harlin MC, Crawford F, Houlden H et al. Early-onset Alzheimer's disease caused by mutations at codon 717 of the β-amyloid precursor protein gene. *Nature* 1991; 353: 844–6.
(6) Brion J-P, Passareiro J-P, Nunez J, Flament-Durand J. Mise en évidence immunologique de la protéine tau an niveau des lésions de dégénérescence neurofibrillaire de la maladie d'Alzheimer. *Arch Biol (Bruxelles)* 1985; 95: 229–35.
(7) Kosik KS, Joachim CL, Selkoe DJ. Microtubule-associated protein tau (τ) is a major antigenic component of paired helical filaments in Alzheimer's disease. *Proc Nat Acad Sci USA* 1986; 83: 4044–8.
(8) Wood JG, Mirra SS, Pollock NJ, Binder LI. Neurofibrillary tangles of Alzheimer's disease share antigenic determinants with the axonal microtubule-associated protein tau (τ). *Proc Nat Acad Sci USA* 1986; 83: 4040–3.
(9) Grundke-Iqbal I, Iqbal K, Quinlan M, Tung YC, Zaidi MS, Wisniewski HM. Microtubule-associated protein tau. A component of Alzheimer paired helical filaments. *J Biol Chem* 1986; 261: 6084–9.

J-M Gallo

(10) Wischik CM, Novak M, Thogersen HC et al. Isolation of a fragment of tau derived from the core of the Alzheimer paired helical filament. *Proc Nat Acad Sci USA* 1988; 85: 4506–10.

(11) Goedert M, Wischik CM, Crowther RA, Walker JE, Klug A. Cloning and sequencing of the cDNA encoding a core protein of the paired helical filament of Alzheimer disease: identification as the microtubule-associated protein tau. *Proc Nat Acad Sci USA* 1988; 85: 4051–5.

(12) Lee G, Cowan N, Kirschner M. The primary structure and heterogeneity of tau protein from mouse brain. *Science* 1988; 239: 285–8.

(13) Kondo J, Honda T, Mori H et al. The carboxyl third of tau is tightly bound to paired helical filaments. *Neuron* 1988; 1: 827–34.

(14) Greenberg SG, Davies P. A preparation of Alzheimer paired helical filaments that displays distinct τ proteins by polyacrylamide gel electrophoresis. *Proc Nat Acad Sci USA* 1990; 87: 5827–31.

(15) Hanger DP, Brion JP, Gallo J-M, Cairns NJ, Luthert PJ, Anderton BH. Tau in Alzheimer's disease and Down's syndrome is insoluble and abnormally phosphorylated. *Biochem J* 1991; 275: 99–104.

(16) Goedert M, Spillantini MG, Cairns NJ, Crowther RA. Tau proteins of Alzheimer paired helical filaments: abnormal phosphorylation of all six brain isoforms. *Neuron* 1992; 8: 159–68.

(17) Flament S, Delacourte A, Hémon B, Défossez A. Evidence biochimique directe d'une phosphorylation anormale des protéines tau durant la maladie d'Alzheimer. *C R Acad Sci (Paris)* 1989; 308: 77–82.

(18) Flament S, Delacourte A. Abnormal tau species are produced during Alzheimer's disease neurodegenerating process. *FEBS Lett* 1989; 247: 213–16.

(19) Flament S, Delacourte A, Hémon B, Défossez A. Characterization of two pathological tau protein variants in Alzheimer brain cortices. *J Neurol Sci* 1989; 92: 133–41.

(20) Goedert M, Spillantini MG, Potier MC, Ulrich J, Crowther RA. Cloning and sequencing of the cDNA encoding an isoform of microtubule-associated protein tau containing four tandem repeats: differential expression of tau protein mRNAs in human brain. *EMBO J* 1989; 8: 393–9.

(21) Goedert M, Spillantini MG, Jakes R, Rutherford D, Crowther RA. Multiple isoforms of human microtubule-associated protein tau: sequences and localization in neurofibrillary tangles of Alzheimer's disease. *Neuron* 1989; 3: 519–26.

(22) Goedert M, Jakes R. Expression of separate isoforms of human tau protein: correlation with the tau pattern in brain and effects on tubulin polymerization. *EMBO J* 1990; 9: 4225–30.

(23) Lee G, Neve RL, Kosik KS. The microtubule binding domain of tau protein. *Neuron* 1989; 2: 1615–24.

(24) Kosik KS, Orecchio LD, Binder L, Trojanowski JQ, Lee VM-L, Lee G. Epitopes that span the tau molecule are shared with paired helical filaments. *Neuron* 1988; 1: 817–25.

(25) Brion J-P, Hanger DP, Bruce MT, Couck A-M, Flament-Durand J, Anderton BH. Tau in Alzheimer neurofibrillary tangles. N- and C-terminal regions are

differentially associated with paired helical filaments and the location of a putative abnormal phosphorylation site. *Biochem J* 1991; 273: 127–33.

(26) Jakes R, Novak M, Davison M, Wischik CM. Identification of 3- and 4-repeat tau isoforms within the PHF in Alzheimer's disease. *EMBO J* 1991; 10: 2725–9.

(27) Brion J-P, Hanger DP, Couck A-M, Anderton BH. A68 proteins in Alzheimer's disease are composed of several tau isoforms in a phosphorylated state which affects their electrophoretic mobilities. *Biochem J* 1991; 279: 831–6.

(28) Ksiezak-Reding H, Liu W-K, Hradsky J, Yen S-H. Phosphate analysis of different tau preparations from normal and Alzheimer's disease brain. *J Cell Biol* 1990; 111: 435a.

(29) Steiner B, Mandelkow E-M, Biernat J et al. Phosphorylation of microtubule-associated protein tau: identification of a site for Ca^{2+}-calmodulin dependent kinase and relationship with tau phosphorylation in Alzheimer tangles. *EMBO J* 1990; 9: 3539–44.

(30) Litersky JM, Johnson GVW. Phosphorylation of tau by cAMP-dependent protein kinase inhibits the degradation of tau by calpain. *J Biol Chem* 1992; 267: 1563–8.

(31) Hanger DP, Loviny TLF, Robertson J, Goedert M, Murray KJ, Anderton BH. Cyclic AMP-dependent protein kinase induces a shift in the electrophoretic mobility of human tau. *Neurobiol Aging* 1992; 13: S54.

(32) Hirokawa N, Shiomura Y, Okabe S. Tau proteins: the molecular structure and mode of binding to microtubules. *J Cell Biol* 1988; 107: 1449–59.

(33) Hagestedt T, Lichtenberg B, Wille H, Mandelkow E-M, Mandelkow E. Tau protein becomes long and stiff upon phosphorylation: correlation between paracrystalline structure and degree of phosphorylation. *J Cell Biol* 1989; 109: 1643–51.

(34) Binder LI, Frankfurter A, Rebhun LI. The distribution of tau in the mammalian central nervous system. *J Cell Biol* 1985; 101: 1371–8.

(35) Grundke-Iqbal I, Iqbal K, Tung YC, Quinlan M, Wisniewski HM, Binder LI. Abnormal phosphorylation of the microtubule-associated protein τ (tau) in Alzheimer cytoskeletal pathology. *Proc Nat Acad Sci USA* 1986; 83: 4913–17.

(36) Biernat J, Mandelkow E-M, Schröter C et al. The switch of tau protein to an Alzheimer-like state includes the phosphorylation of two serine-proline motifs upstream of the microtubule binding region. *EMBO J* 1992; 11: 1593–7.

(37) Lee VM-Y, Balin BJ, Otvos L, Trojanowski JQ. A68: A major subunit of paired helical filaments and derivatized form of normal tau. *Science* 1991; 251: 675–9.

(38) Iqbal K, Grundke-Iqbal I, Smith AJ, George L, Tung Y-C, Zaidi T. Identification and localization of a τ peptide to paired helical filaments of Alzheimer's disease. *Proc Nat Acad Sci USA* 1989; 86: 5646–50.

(39) Anderton BH, Breinburg D, Downes MJ et al. Monoclonal antibodies show that neurofibrillary tangles and neurofilaments share antigenic determinants. *Nature* 1982; 298: 84–6.

(40) Sternberger NH, Sternberger LA, Ulrich J. Aberrant neurofilament phosphorylation in Alzheimer's disease. *Proc Nat Acad Sci USA* 1985; 82: 4274–6.

(41) Lee VM-Y, Otvos LJr, Schmidt ML, Trojanowski JQ. Alzheimer's disease tangles share immunological similarities with multiphosphorylation repeats in the two large neurofilament proteins. *Proc Nat Acad Sci USA* 1988; 85: 7384–8.

(42) Coleman MP, Anderton BH. Phosphate-dependent monoclonal antibodies to neurofilaments and Alzheimer neurofibrillary tangles recognize a synthetic phosphopeptide. *J Neurochem* 1990; 54: 1548–55.

(43) Sternberger NH, Sternberger LA. Monoclonal antibodies distinguish phosphorylated and nonphosphorylated forms of neurofilaments in situ. *Proc Nat Acad Sci USA* 1983; 80: 6126–30.

(44) Lichtenberg-Kraag B, Mandelkow E-M, Biernat J et al. Phosphorylation-dependent epitopes of neurofilament antibodies on tau protein and relationship with Alzheimer tau. *Proc Nat Acad Sci USA* 1992; 89: 5384–8.

(45) Drewes G, Lichtenberg-Kraag B, Döring F et al. Mitogen activated protein (MAP) kinase transforms tau protein into an Alzheimer-like state. *EMBO J* 1992; 11: 2131–8.

(46) Roder HM, Ingram VM. Two novel kinases phosphorylate tau and the KSP site of heavy neurofilament subunits in high stoichiometric ratios. *J Neurosci* 1991; 11: 3325–43.

(47) Ishiguro K, Ihara Y, Uchida T, Imahori K. A novel tubulin-dependent protein kinase forming a paired helical filament epitope on tau. *J Biochem (Tokyo)* 1988; 104: 319–21.

(48) Ishiguro K, Omori A, Sato K, Tomizawa K, Imahori K, Uchida T. A serine/threonine proline kinase activity is included in the tau protein kinase fraction forming a paired helical filament epitope. *Neurosci Lett* 1991; 128: 195–8.

(49) Ishiguro K, Takamatsu M, Tomizawa K et al. Tau protein kinase I converts normal tau protein into A68-like component of paired helical filaments. *J Biol Chem* 1992; 267: 10897–901.

(50) Wolozin BL, Pruchnicki A, Dickson DW, Davies P. A neuronal antigen in the brains of Alzheimer patients. *Science* 1986; 232: 648–50.

(51) Ksiezak-Reding H, Binder LI, Yen S-H. Immunochemical and biochemical characterization of τ proteins in normal and Alzheimer's disease brains with Alz 50 and Tau-1. *J Biol Chem* 1988; 263: 7943–53.

(52) Nukina N, Kosik KS, Selkoe DJ. The monoclonal antibody, Alz 50, recognizes tau proteins in Alzheimer's disease brain. *Neurosci Lett* 1988; 87: 240–6.

(53) Hyman BT, Van Hoesen GW, Wolozin BL, Davies P, Kromer LJ, Damasio AR. Alz-50 antibody recognizes Alzheimer-related neuronal changes. *Ann Neurol* 1988; 23: 371–9.

(54) Ksiezak-Reding H, Chien C-H, Lee VM-Y, Yen S-H. Mapping of the Alz 50 epitope in microtubule-associated proteins tau. *J Neurosci Res* 1990; 25: 412–19.

(55) Uéda K, Masliah E, Saitoh T, Bakalis SL, Scoble H, Kosik KS. Alz-50 recognizes a phosphorylated epitope of tau protein. *J Neurosci* 1990; 10: 3295–304.

(56) Vincent IJ, Davies P. A protein kinase associated with paired helical filaments in Alzheimer's disease. *Proc Nat Acad Sci USA* 1992; 89: 2878–82.

(57) Goedert M, Spillantini MG, Jakes R. Localization of the Alz-50 epitope in recombinant human microtubule-associated protein tau. *Neurosci Lett* 1991; 126: 149–54.

(58) Mori H, Kondo J, Ihara Y. Ubiquitin is a component of paired helical filaments in Alzheimer's disease. *Science* 1987; 235: 1641–4.

(59) Gallo J-M, Anderton BH. Ubiquitous variations in nerves. *Nature* 1989; 337: 687–8.

(60) Brion J-P, Power D, Hue D, Couck AM, Anderton BH, Flament-Durand J. Heterogeneity of ubiquitin immunoreactivity in neurofibrillary tangles of Alzheimer's disease. *Neurochem Int* 1989; 14: 121–8.

(61) Perry G, Mulvihill P, Fried VA, Smith HT, Grundke-Iqbal I, Iqbal K. Immunochemical properties of ubiquitin conjugates in the paired helical filaments of Alzheimer's disease. *J Neurochem* 1989; 52: 1523–8.

(62) Grundke-Iqbal I, Vorbrodt AW, Iqbal K, Tung Y-C, Wang GP, Wisniewski HM. Microtubule-associated polypeptides tau are altered in Alzheimer paired helical filaments. *Molec Brain Res* 1988; 4: 43–52.

(63) Vincent IJ, Davies P. ATP-induced loss of Alz-50 immunoreactivity with the A68 proteins from Alzheimer brain is mediated by ubiquitin. *Proc Nat Acad Sci USA* 1990; 87: 4840–4.

(64) Lindwall G, Cole RD. Phosphorylation affects the ability of tau to promote microtubule assembly. *J Biol Chem* 1984; 259: 5301–5.

(65) Nieto A, Correas I, López-Otín C, Avila J. Tau-related protein present in paired helical filaments has a decreased tubulin binding capacity as compared with microtubule-associated protein tau. *Biochem Biophys Acta* 1991; 1096: 197–204.

(66) Caceres A, Kosik KS. Inhibition of neurite polarity by tau antisense oligonucleotides in primary cerebellar neurons. *Nature* 1990; 343: 461–3.

(67) Caceres A, Potrebic S, Kosik KS. The effect of tau antisense oligonucleotides on neurite formation of cultured cerebellar macroneurons. *J Neurosci* 1991; 11: 1515–23.

(68) Mattson MP. Effect of microtubule stabilization and destabilization on tau immunoreactivity in cultured hippocampal neurons. *Brain Res* 1992; 582: 107–18.

(69) Lantos PL, Luthert PJ, Hanger D, Anderton BH, Mullan M, Rossor M. Familial Alzheimer's disease with the amyloid precursor protein position 717 mutation and sporadic Alzheimer's disease have the same cytoskeletal pathology. *Neurosci Lett* 1992; 137: 221–4.

(70) Flament S, Delacourte A, Mann DMA. Phosphorylation of tau proteins: a major event during the process of neurofibrillary degeneration. A comparative study between Alzheimer's disease and Down's syndrome. *Brain Res* 1990; 516: 15–19.

(71) Frautschy SA, Baird A, Cole GM. Effects of injected Alzheimer β-amyloid cores in rat brain. *Proc Nat Acad Sci USA* 1991; 88: 8362–6.

(72) Kowal NW, Beal MF, Busciglio J, Duffy LK, Yankner BA. An in vivo model for the neurodegenerative effects of β amyloid and protection by substance P. *Proc Nat Acad Sci USA* 1991; 88: 7247–51.

(73) Maruyama K, Terakado K, Usami M, Yoshikawa K. Formation of amyloid-like fibrils in COS cells overexpressing part of the Alzheimer amyloid protein precursor. *Nature* 1990; 347: 566–9.

(74) Yankner BA, Davies LR, Fisher S, Villa-Kmaroff L, Oster-Granite ML, Neve

RL. Neurotoxicity of a fragment of the amyloid precursor associated with Alzheimer's disease. *Science* 1989; 245: 417–20.

(75) Neve RL, Kammesheidt A, Hohmann CF. Brain transplants of cells expressing the carboxyl-terminal fragment of the Alzheimer amyloid protein precursor cause specific neuropathology. *Proc Nat Acad Sci USA* 1992; 89: 3448–52.

(76) Koh J-Y, Yang LL, Cotman CW. β-Amyloid protein increases the vulnerability of cultured cortical neurons to excitotoxic damage. *Brain Res* 1990; 533: 315–20.

(77) Mattson MP, Cheng B, Davis D, Bryant K, Lieberburg I, Rydel RE. β-amyloid peptides destabilize calcium homeostasis and render human cortical neurons vulnerable to excitotoxicity. *J Neurosci* 1992; 12: 376–89.

(78) Mattson MP. Antigenic changes similar to those seen in neurofibrillary tangles are elicited by glutamate and Ca^{2+} influx in cultured hippocampal neurons. *Neuron* 1990; 4: 105–17.

Cytoarchitectonic and developmental studies in schizophrenia

P FALKAI and B BOGERTS

Historical considerations

Kraepetin was one of the first to believe in the neuropathological basis of schizophrenia. In his clinic in Munich, he gathered together people such as Alzheimer, Gaup and Nissl to investigate the brains of patients suffering from schizophrenia. Alzheimer was one of the first to publish an article, in which he described pallor and loss of cells in the neocortex of schizophrenics[1]. Subsequently, about 200 papers were published until 1952, when at the 'First International Congress of Neuropathology in Rome' internationally acknowledged neuropathologists tried to find the common substrate of schizophrenia. Not being able to do so, they concluded that the brains of patients with schizophrenia show no abnormality which could be attributed specifically to the disease process.

After the failure of classical neuropathological schizophrenia research to demonstrate convincingly anatomical anomalies in the brains of schizophrenics, a new era of pathomorphological interest in schizophrenia received strong impetus from an article published by Stevens[2] postulating morphological changes in limbic and basal ganglia structures, and was prompted by modern neuroimaging techniques such as computed tomography (CT) and magnetic resonance imaging (MRI).

Here we review the development of neuropathological schizophrenia research during the last 20 years. For earlier studies, several comprehensive reviews exist[3-5]. Recent interest in the neuroanatomy of schizophrenia has focused on brain size and weight, the limbic system with its important telencephalic components comprising the medial temporal lobe structures and the cingulate gyrus, the prefrontal cortex, the basal ganglia, and most importantly the globus pallidus, the corpus callosum, and the thalamus.

All correspondence to: Dr P Falkai, Neurohistological Laboratory, Department of Psychiatry, University of Düsseldorf, Bergische Landstraße 2, 4000 Düsseldorf 1, Germany.

Cambridge Medical Reviews: Neurobiology and Psychiatry Volume 2
© Cambridge University Press

P Falkai and B Bogerts

Regions of interest

Brain size and brain weight

Postmortem results on brain weight and brain size are conflicting. While some early poorly controlled studies did not find cerebral atrophy or reduced brain weight[6], others described qualitatively cerebral atrophy in a significant percentage of the patients[4,7]. Three recent controlled quantitative studies found significant decreases in brain weight by 5–8%[8–10] and significant reductions (4%) of brain anterior–posterior length[10], while one study found nearly identical brain weight and hemispheric volumes in schizophrenics and controls[11].

Temporolimbic structures

Since the first report of reduced tissue volume in temporolimbic structures of schizophrenics 10 years ago[12], some 25 quantitative or qualitative anatomical postmortem studies in limbic structures of schizophrenics have been published. Of these studies, 21 found subtle structural changes in at least one of the investigated areas[8,13–33], whereas three yielded entirely negative results[34–36]. The findings comprise reduced volumes or cross-sectional areas of the hippocampus, amygdala and parahippocampal gyrus[8,13–15,18,20,22,23,25], which were later corroborated by morphometric MRI studies of mesiotemporal structures[37–45]. Other findings in limbic brain regions are: left temporal horn enlargement[8,14,24], reduced cell numbers or cell size in hippocampus or parahippocampal gyrus/entorhinal cortex[17,18,20,23,26,30], white matter reductions in parahippocampal gyrus or hippocampus[22,33], disturbed cytoarchitecture, increased vertical axon numbers, and deficits in small interneurons in the cingulate gyrus[27,28,30,46], abnormal cell arrangements in the hippocampus or entorhinal cortex[16,17,19,21,31,32], and an increased incidence of a cavum septi pellucidi[47].

Two groups could not confirm cellular disarray in the hippocampus[30,34], and one group could not find significant volume and cell number reductions in the hippocampus and entorhinal cortex[33,35,36].

Although the type and extent of the reported limbic system pathology vary, and although there is no homogenous pattern of limbic pathology in schizophrenia, the vast majority of the authors agree that there are subtle changes in limbic brain regions in a significant percentage of schizophrenics. The extent of the pathology is not comparable by far to that seen in the known degenerative brain diseases. Limbic tissue volumes, cell numbers and size differ by some 10–30% between schizophrenics and controls, and there is a considerable overlap between patients and controls, about one-quarter of the patients having values outside the range of the controls.

Cortex

As already mentioned, nearly 100 years ago, Alzheimer[1] described pallor and loss of pyramidal cells in the cortex of patients with dementia precox. Some years later, Southard[48] reported atrophy mainly in the cortical association centres. In the new era of neuropathological schizophrenia research, very few histopathological studies of the cortex have been performed. There are reports of a reduction of cortical thickness and cell loss in deep cortical layers[49], lower neuronal densities and deficits in small interneurons in the prefrontal cortex and anterior cingulate gyrus[29,50].

Three planimetric postmortem studies of the whole cortex have been performed: one reported significant reductions of cortical volume (12%) and central grey (6%)[9], the two others reported virtually identical volumes of cortex, white matter and whole hemispheres in schizophrenics and controls[11,51].

Basal ganglia

Unchanged volumes of the striatum and external pallidum, but a subtle volume decrease in the internal pallidal segment, were found in brains from the preneuroleptic era[58]. Pallidal volume reduction was due to a reduction in the catatonic subgroup[53,139]. In the same brains, catatonics had a decreased diameter of the microneurons in the striatum[54]. A study of patients chronically treated with neuroleptics found bilaterally increased striatal volumes reaching a significant level on the left side[38]. It is remarkable that two MRI studies also found larger striatal volumes or cross-sectional areas in chronically treated schizophrenics[45,55]. Since it is known that neuroleptics cause a functional hyperactivity of the striatum owing to a blockade of inhibitory dopaminergic input, it is possible that long term neuroleptic treatment leads to an activation hypertrophia of the striatum.

Data from qualitative[56,57] and quantitative postmortem studies[53,58], as well as from recent brain perfusion studies[59,60], support the notion that pallidal dysfunction might occur in catatonic schizophrenics. Catatonia is characterized by abnormal movements combined with positive as well as with negative symptoms. Striatum and pallidum are regarded as being parts of the extrapyramidal and limbic system[61] and are involved in the neuronal modulation of movement coordination. It is therefore conceivable that dysfunction of these brain parts plays a role in the pathogenesis of catatonic symptoms.

Corpus callosum

Structural anomalies of the midline area of the corpus callosum were demonstrated by several MRI scan and postmortem studies[51,62–68,138]. The findings, however, are inconsistent; there are reports of increased[51] as well as of decreased[66,67] midline areas. More consistent are reports of shape abnormalities, in that the sex difference in anterior and posterior callosal thickness in normal controls seems to be reversed in schizophrenics[62,63], and the mean curvature in the corpus callosum is more marked in schizophrenics[46], with the corpus callosum being thicker in female schizophrenics and thinner in male schizophrenics.

Thalamus

Cell loss and reduced tissue volume of medial thalamic structures had already been described several decades ago in schizophrenics of the Vogt collection[69-71]. although two studies investigating the same brain material as did the earlier studies[54,72] failed to replicate these findings, one controlled morphometric investigation using another brain collection has again found volume and cell number reductions similar to those reported in the original studies in the mediodorsal nucleus of the thalamus[73].

If thalamic dysfunction caused schizophrenia-like symptoms, as assumed by some authors[74,75], such a symptomatology might be expected in patients with known organic diseases of the thalamus. In the quite extensive literature on organic lesions of the thalamus and diencephalon, clinical symptoms such as apathy, drowsiness, mental lethargy, stuporous conditions, disturbances of memory, and sensory phenomena such as hypasthesia, hyperpathia, and painful perceptions are described as being most characteristic[72]. Positive psychotic symptoms usually do not occur. Thus clinical symptoms associated with dysfunction of the thalamus resemble the negative symptoms of schizophrenia. This assumption is supported by the observation that, in CT scans of schizophrenics, third ventricular enlargement (possibly indicating atrophy of the surrounding thalamus) occurs in patients with chronic negative symptoms[76].

Brain stem neurotransmitter systems

Two qualitative reports on degenerative changes in the cholinergic basal nucleus of schizophrenics have been published[77]; a more recent quantitative study found normal cell numbers in the basal nucleus of schizophrenics[78].

The lateral (nigrostriatal) and medial (mesolimbic) parts of the mesencephalic dopaminergic systems of six chronic schizophrenics (six controls) were evaluated by Bogerts et al.[94]. There was a significant volume reduction by about 21% of the lateral parts of the substantia nigra, and the size of the nerve cell bodies was significantly reduced in the medial part by 16%. Cell numbers were unchanged. The reduced cell size of the medial, mesolimbic neurons was taken as indicative of a dopaminergic underactivity rather than an overactivity of these cells in the schizophrenics investigated.

Lohr and Jeste[79] undertook volume measurements and cell counts in the noradrenergic locus coeruleus of 15 schizophrenics of the Yakovlev collection. There was a trend for decreased locus coeruleus volume without loss of neurons, indicating a reduction of neuropil in the schizophrenics as compared to leucotomized controls. The results appeared comparable to those described in the substantia nigra[94].

Investigating the brain stem reticular formation in four patients as compared to five controls, Karson et al.[80] found a twofold *increased* number of cholinergic neurons of the pedunculopontine nucleus and of the dorsal tegmental nucleus as well as a reduced cell size in the locus coeruleus.

Possible clues to mechanisms underlying the neuropathological changes

Gliosis

The glial elements of the central nervous system include the neuroglia and the microglia. The neuroglia, sometimes known as macroglia, consist of the astrocytes, oligodendroglia and ependymal cells. The astrocytes form the majority and are classified as protoplasmic or fibrous forms, the former being largely confined to grey matter, and the latter to white matter. Although astrocytes clearly play a structurally supportive role in the nervous system, there may be specialized subclasses of astrocytes performing different functions : (i) guidance of migrating neurons to their permanent positions in the cortex[82,83]; (ii) insulating role[84]; (iii) regulation of the ionic composition of extracellular fluid, eg reducing the extracellular K^+ concentration after neural activation[85] or taking up neurotransmitters like GABA, glutamate and amines[86]; and (iv) reaction of injury (= reactive gliosis).

Astrocytes show changes in response to almost every type of injury or disease in the central nervous system[81]. This may take the form of degeneration, hypertrophy or hyperplasia. The capacity of astrocytes to react with proliferation and hypertrophy develops during the last trimester of gestation, and is already evident in the mature newborn[87]. Astrocytosis is not a static process but rather one that evolves with time[88]. Immediately after injury, astrocytes undergo both hyperplasia and hypertrophy in an attempt to repair the damage. These plump cellular elements stain with the glial fibrillary acid protein (GFAP) antibody. As the tissue repair response matures, astrocytic bodies diminish in number while their fibrils become more prominent. The resultant chronic fibrillary gliosis is best detected by special stains such as the Holzer technique[81,91]. From the point of view of the chronic progressive course of schizophrenia in a subset of patients, it is interesting to note that, in conditions such as subacute sclerosing panencephalitis, the evidence for neuronal loss is not readily seen but the astrocytes form pairs or groups indicating previous cell death. In addition, in a chronic, slowly progressive condition such as leucodystrophy, the astrocytic cells may only be markedly enlarged but their number not increased[81].

From about 50 postmortem studies published in the last 20 years on schizophrenia, 18 specifically addressed the question of gliosis. What information can we get out of them?

Fibrous gliosis Applying stains for glial fibres like Holzer staining, glial knots in the brainstem[89], diffuse gliosis in the diencephalon, mesencephalon and hippocampus[91] and fibrous gliosis in the hypothalamus, midbrain tegmentum, bed nucleus of the stria terminalis, basal nucleus, medial thalamus, amygdala and hippocampus[57] were described. Examining all brain regions, no evidence for gliosis using Holzer stain was found in a brain sample, where cases with focal pathology were excluded[10].

Glial cell counts (astrocytes and oligodendroglia) Using GFAP-staining, three studies failed to find a significant increase in astrocytes using densiometry[91,92] and manual cell counts[93] in temporal lobe structures. Astroglial cell densities were unchanged in the anterior cingulate and prefrontal cortex[20]. An assay of diazepam-binding inhibitor-like immunoreactivity was applied in one study, parallel to using the Holzer technique in the contralateral hemisphere, but neither technique showed a difference between groups in any brain region[24]. Glial cells in general were determined on Nissl stained sections in five studies. No significant difference between schizophrenics and controls for glial cell densities or absolute glial counts could be detected in the mesencephalon[94], prefrontal, anterior cingulate and primary motor cortex[50], the corpus callosum[62], the hippocampus[18] and the entorhinal cortex[20]. The density of astrocytes and oligodendroglia was reduced in the mediodorsal thalamic nucleus and in the nucleus accumbens, but unchanged in the ventral pallidum and basolateral nucleus of the amygdala[73].

Neuron–glia ratio The neuron–glia ratios for each layer of the prefrontal, anterior cingulate and primary motor cortex were calculated but showed no difference between schizophrenics and controls[50].

Volume of glial cell nuclei Numerical densities, absolute numbers and average volume of melanin containing dopaminergic neurons of the nigrostriatal system and of the mesolimbic system were carried out on Nissl stained serial sections of nine normal brains, six age matched brains of schizophrenics, five brains of paralysis agitans, and six brains of postencephalitic Parkinsonism. The average volume of the glial cell nuclei was significantly smaller in schizophrenics compared to control subjects in the nigrostriatal system and tended to be smaller in the limbic system[94].

In summary, studies using glial cell counts, neuron–glial ratios and glial cell nuclei volumes showed no difference between schizophrenics and controls. Three out of four studies using glial fibre stains showed a significant increase of glial fibres in schizophrenics. In a very elegant study, also using

Holzer stain, Casanova and coworkers quantified the number of astrocytic markers within the terminal fields of the perforant pathway originating from the entorhinal cortex in schizophrenics, in patients with Alzheimer's disease, and in healthy control subjects. Half of the patients with Alzheimer's disease had astrocytosis in the terminal fields of the perforant pathway, which is the dentate region of the hippocampus. There was an absence of similar changes in the schizophrenic group, and the authors concluded that such a lesion in the entorhinal cortex is therefore static in nature and occurred many years before the patients were autopsied[95]. These data and the well controlled study of Bruton et al.[10] reject fibrous gliosis in schizophrenia. However, there is evidence from follow up studies, that at least a subgroup of chronically deteriorating patients show progressive lesions in the CT scan[96]. Therefore it seems unlikely that the majority of schizophrenic patients show a considerable degree of gliosis, but there might be a small subgroup showing gliotic changes.

Remnants of disturbed neurodevelopment

There are three stages, or life cycles, in the embryonic development of the cellular elements of the cerebral cortex, and there are three corresponding morphogenetic fields where these cellular transformations take place[97].

1. Growth of a large pool of proliferative precursor cells of neurons and glia. This takes place in the germinal matrix (primarily in the neuro-epithelium and to a lesser extent, the subventricular zone) of the cortical primordium.
2. Translocation of differentiating cells in to the intermediate zone. The migrating young neurons begin to sprout their axons before they proceed toward the surface of the cortex.
3. Settling of neurons in the future cerebral cortex, composed of the primordial plexiform layer and the cortical plate. It is at the latter sites that the final differentiation of neurons, including their dendritic development and synaptic organization, takes place.

The gravest structural anomalies, in general, result from disorders that disrupt cytogenetic or histogenetic events. Among these, survival is improbable and, where it occurs, functional disability is grave. Substantial disability may result from disorders of development which do not lead to deformities that are grossly evident at birth. Large numbers of these lesser disturbances may be ascertained only by their functional consequences, such as disturbances of learning, language disorders, autism, and recurrent seizures. It is probable that these milder disorders reflect, in most instances, disturbances of the processes of growth and differentiation[98].

Subtle cytoarchitectural anomalies were described in the hippocampal formation[16,32,99,100], frontal cortex, cingulate gyrus[27,50] and entorhinal cortex[17,19,21,31] in patients suffering from schizophrenia compared to control subjects.

McLardy found a significant thinning of the granular layer of the dentate gyrus in 30% of schizophrenic patients, 100% of chronic alcoholics, and in none of the controls. The cell picture in schizophrenia did not have a degenerative appearance, but was fully consistent with developmental arrest[99].

Qualitatively, and later quantitatively, a significant cellular disarray in the CA3/CA4 interface was described in the left[16,100] and replicated in the right hippocampus[32]. This was interpreted as a bilateral migrational abnormality and broadly correlated with the degree of disease severity. Altshuler et al.[101] were not able to fully replicate the study, but did confirm a within case correlation with severity; whereas Christison et al.[34] did not find a significant disarray distinguishing schizophrenics from controls.

On Nissl stained sections, the neuronal density was significantly lower in layer VI of the prefrontal, layer V of the cingulate, and in layer III of the motor cortex[50]. In a subsequent study, clusters of cells were found in the anterior cingulate cortex of schizophrenic patients, which were smaller in size and separated by wider distances than those observed in the controls group[27]. This finding was supported by a 25% increase of vertical axons in schizophrenics in the cingulate cortex[28].

An abnormal sulcogyral pattern or abnormal gross configuration of the temporal lobe and cytoarchitectonic abnormalities of the rostral entorhinal region as well as of the ventral insular cortex of schizophrenics were described recently[17,102]. The cytoarchitectonic abnormalities of the rostral entorhinal region consisted of heterotopic pre-alpha cells in the pre beta layer (= third layer), which would normally belong to the pre-alpha layer (= second layer).

Rating abnormally positioned (heterotopic) pre-alpha cell clusters in the entorhinal cortex, we found a significant increase of the mean rating values in schizophrenics on the left side of 43% ($p < .03$). Patients with a family history of psychiatric illness compared to schizophrenics without such a history had significantly more heterotopic clusters on the left side ($+49\%$, $p < .01$), but were no different on the right side. There was a trend for an inversive correlation between onset of the disease and the heterotopic ratings in the left entorhinal cortex ($r = -.298$; $p < .10$), suggesting that earlier onset of the disease is associated with more heterotopias in the left entorhinal cortex[103]. In conclusion, cytoarchitectonic abnormalities recently described in different limbic structures in schizophrenia are very subtle and will easily be missed using classical neuropathological methods. Quantifying them often needs sophisticated staining methods, eg immunohistochemistry[28], serial sections and a matched control group. It is unlikely that the subtle differences found are due to disturbances in the proliferative or early migrational phase, but rather are caused by disturbances in late migration or in final differentiation of neurons. The misplaced neurons in the entorhinal cortex, for instance, could be a sign of disturbed late neuronal migration, or could mirror disturbed programmed cell death, as heterotopias are frequently found in the temporal cortex of autopsied children, which seem to disappear in adults[104].

Left/right differences: reversed or reduced asymmetry?

Since 1972, more than 50 postmortem studies on schizophrenia have been published, of which 22 examined both brain hemispheres. Of these 22 studies, 8 found changes on the left, 2 on the right, 5 bilaterally and in 7 there were either negative findings or it was not clear from the publication which hemisphere was meant (for further details see Tables 1–3). Four studies[8,21,24,103] examined diagnosis by side interactions, and three[8,21,24] found a significant interaction for the left hemisphere. There is a growing number of MRI studies supporting the notion of an increased prevalence of left hemispheric pathology in schizophrenia, eg Bogerts et al.[52]. He found a significant volume reduction of the left hippocampus accompanied by a significant volume increase of the left temporal horn in first break schizophrenia. Is there a common mechanism possibly causing left lateralized changes in the brains of schizophrenic patients?

In a recent study, Crow et al.[24] filled the lateral ventricle of half brains of 56 schizophrenics, 56 matched control subjects and 30 patients with Alzheimer's disease with radiopaque material. A roentgenographic image of the ventricle from the lateral aspect was then obtained. To define the location of the brain changes, the area of the anterior horn, the body and the posterior and temporal horns of ventricle were determined. In Alzheimer-type dementia, there was a relatively uniform increase in the area of the ventricular components. In schizophrenia, the size of the posterior and particularly of the temporal horn was increased (by 28% and 82%, respectively). Diagnosis by side interaction revealed a selective enlargement of the left temporal horn in schizophrenia compared to the control group. Excluding all brains with neuropathological signs of significant disease, the brains of 22 schizophrenics and 26 controls were reanalysed, giving the same result. Using Holzer stain and diazepam binding inhibitor immunoreactivity, no significant increase of glial fibre/cell densities was obtained in the purified series. The authors concluded that these findings are consistent with the view that schizophrenia is a disorder of the genetic mechanism that controls the development of cerebral asymmetry.

To prove the hypothesis that cerebral asymmetry is disturbed in schizophrenia, we examined the Sylvian fissure and planum temporale in two subsequent postmortem studies. Both structures belong to the most asymmetrical anatomical areas in the human brain, are usually longer/bigger in the left compared to the right hemisphere and seem to represent the morphological correlate for lateralized functions in man, eg language and handedness.

51

Table 1. *Findings pointing at disturbed brain development*

Authors	Number of patients (and controls)	Hemisphere examined	Findings with reference to hemisphere	Side × diagnosis interaction
McLardy[99]	30 (7)	No comment	Reduced thickness of the granule cell layer in the hippocampal formation without degeneration appearance	–
Scheibel & Kovelman[100]	10(8)	Left	Disorientation of hippocampal pyramidal cells	–
Bogerts et al.[13, 58]	13(10)	Left	Reduced volumes of hippocampus, parahippocampal gyrus and amygdala (Vogt collection)	–
Kovelman & Scheibel[16]	10(8)	Left	Disarray of hippocampal pyramidal cells	–
Benes et al.[28, 50]	10(10)	No comment	Reduced neuronal density without gliosis, cytoarchitectural disturbances in the prefrontal cortex, anterior cingulate and primary motor cortex	–
Falkai & Bogerts[18]	13(11)	Left	Reduction of hippocampal pyramidal cells without gliosis	–

Study	n	Hemisphere	Findings	
Benes et al.[29]	14(9)	No comment	Reduced pyramidal cell density in CA1 segment in schizophrenics with mood disorder, overall reduction of pyramidal cell size	—
Benes et al.[30]	18(12)	No comment	Reduction of interneurons in layer II of the cingulate and the prefrontal cortex, reduced number of pyramidal cells in layer V of prefrontal region	—
Jakob & Beckmann[17]	64(10)	Left + right	Cytoarchitectonic abnormalities in the rostral entorhinal region, abnormal pattern of temporal sulci with a preference of the left hemisphere	—
Brown et al.[8]	41(29)	Left + right	Reduction of brain weight, bilateral reduction of parahippocampal thickness, ventricular, especially temporal horn enlargment bilaterally	Left parahippocampal cortex
Roberts et al.[91]	12(12)	Left	No significant difference of astrocyte densities in the temporal lobe of schizophrenics	—
Roberts et al.[92]	18(20)	Left + right	No significant difference of astrocyte densities in the temporal lobe between schizophrenics, affectives and control subjects	—

Table 1. *Findings pointing at disturbed brain development (cont.)*

Authors	Number of patients (and controls)	Hemisphere examined	Findings with reference to hemisphere	Side × diagnosis interaction
Altshuler et al.[101]	7(6)	No comment	Correlation between hippocampal pyramidal cell disarray and severity of clinical symptoms	–
Falkai et al.[20]	13(11)	Left	Lower volume and cell densities in the entorhinal cortex without gliosis	–
Jakob & Beckmann[102]	12(12)	Left + right	Disturbed convolutional pattern, cytoarchitectonic abnormalities, in the rostral entorhinal cortex and ventral insular region with a preference of the left hemisphere, normal glial cells	–
Falkai & Bogerts[19]	11(7)	Left	Abnormal location of entorhinal prealpha cell clusters	–
Crow et al.[24]	56(56)	Left + right	Selective left temporal horn enlargement found	Left temporal horn
Bogerts et al.[41]	18(21)	Left + right	Reduced hippocampal volume (new Düsseldorf collection)	–
Altshuler et al.[25]	12(27)	Left or right	Reduced cross-sectional area of right parahippocampal gyrus but not hippocampus; shape abnormalities in medial temporal structures	–

Author	N(N)	Side	Findings	Asymmetry
Pakkenberg et al.[73]	12(12)	Left	Reduction of total neuron and glial cell number in mediodorsal thalamic nucleus and nucleus accumbens	—
Arnold et al.[31]	6(16)	Left + right	Aberrant invaginations of the surface, disruption of cortical layers, heterotopic displacement of neurons, paucity of neurons in superficial layers in the para hippocampal gyrus, no preference of side, no gliosis	—
Conrad et al.[32]	11(7)	Right	Dissary of pyramidal cells in right hippocampus	—
Karson et al.[80]	4(5)	Right	Increase of cholinergic neurons in the nucelus pedunculopontinus, decrease of catecholaminergic neurons in the locus coeruleus	—
Degreef et al.[47]	28(39)	Left + right	Increased prevalence of a cavum septum pellucidum	—
Falkai et al.[103]	35(33)	Left + right	Reduction of left Sylvian fissure length, loss of physiological left/right Sylvian fissure asymmetry	Length of left Sylvian fissure
Falkai et al.[21]	19(21)	Left + right	Increased prevalence of heterotopic prealpha cell clusters in the left entorhinal cortex of schizophrenics, especially patients with a family history or early onset of the disease	Prevalence of heterotopic cells in the left entorhinal cortex

Table 2. Findings pointing at an inflammatory, possibly chronic progressive brain disease

Authors	Number of patients (and controls)	Hemisphere examined	Findings with reference to hemisphere	Side × diagnosis interaction
Nieto & Escobar[90]	10(4)	No comment	Gliosis iin the hippocampus	–
Fisman[89]	10(10)	No comment	Glial knots and and perivascular infiltrations in brainstem	–
Averback[77]	13(35)	Left + right	Cellular degeneration in the nucleus of the ansa lenticularis	– –
Stevens[57]	25(48)	No comment	Hypothalamic gliosis, gliosis in the midbrain tegmentum, bed nucleus of the stria terminalis, basal nucleus, medial thalamus amygdala and hippocampus	–
Bigelow et al.[138]	18(11)	–	Gliosis in late onset schizophrenia compared to early onset schizophrenia (anteriorly and posteriorly)	–
Bruton et al.[10]	56(56)	Left + right	Reduction of brain weight and brain length, increase of ventricular size, periventricular fibrous gliosis in half of the schizophrenic cases	–

Table 3. *Studies not specifically pointing at either etiology*

Authors	Number of patients (and controls)	Hemisphere examined	Findings with reference to hemisphere	Side × diagnosis interaction
Rosenthal & Bigelow[51]	10(10)	Right	Increase in corpus callosum width	–
Dom et al.[54]	5(5)	Left	Reduced microneuron density in the pulvinar of catatonic patients	–
Bogerts et al.[94]	15(12)	Left	Reduced volume of the lateral substania nigra, smaller neurons in A 10 area, mean volume of glial nuclei reduced	–
Lesch & Bogerts[72]	15(12)	Left	Reduction of thickness of periventricular grey matter, unchanged volumes of thalamic subnuclei	–
Colter et al.[22]	17(11)	Left or right	Reduced parahippocampal white matter	–
Pakkenberg[9]	29(30)	Left + right	Volume reduction of both hemispheres, the cortex and subcortical white matter and brain weight,	–

Table 3. *Studies not specifically pointing at either etiology (cont.)*

Authors	Number of patients (and controls)	Hemisphere examined	Findings with reference to hemisphere	Side × diagnosis interaction
Lohr & Jeste[79]	15(15)	Left + right	increased ventricular volume, no comment on side differences Reduced neuropil in the locus	—
Jeste & Lohr[23]	13(26)	Left + right	Coeruleus. Reduction of hippocampal volume and pyramidal cell numbers	—
Christison et al.[34]	14(29)	Left + right	No disarray of hippocampal pyramidal cells	—
Heckers et al.[35]	20(20)	Left + right	Unchanged volume of parahippocampal gyrus	—
Heckers et al.[36]	20(20)	Left + right	Unchanged volume of hippocampus amygdala and ventricular system, significant increase of left ventricular volume in paranoid schizophrenia	—
Heckers et al.[33]	13(13)	Left + right	Reduction of hippo-campal white matter, no differences in	—

| Heckers et al.[11] | 23(23) | Left + right | total cell numbers, cell density and volume of hippocampus, non significant decrease of absolute cell numbers in the left CA1 region Bilateral increase of striatal volume right sided increase of palladal volume, none of white matter and cortex | – |
| Casanova et al.[26] | 8(18) | Left + right | Bilateral reduction of cell counts in the ento-rhinal cortex, no change in cross-sectional area | – |

In the first study, the Sylvian fissure (= SF) length was measured in postmortem brains of 35 schizophrenic patients and 33 matched non-psychiatric control subjects of the New Düsseldorf Brain Collection, Department of Psychiatry. The schizophrenics showed a significantly reduced length of the left SF (-16%, $p < .0001$) compared to the control subjects, while the right SF length was unchanged. SF asymmetry, expressed as left/right SF length ratio, was more reduced in male schizophrenics (-24%, $p < .001$) than in female patients (-16%, $p < .03$)[21]. Recently, a significant ($p < .002$) reduction in brain length, a relative reduction in Sylvian fissure length on the left, and a reduction in the vertical distance between the Sylvian point and the dorsal surface of the brain on the left side, was found replicating the finding mentioned above[106].

As there is a correlation between the area of the planum temporale and the length of the Sylvian fissure[107], we determined in a second study the volume of the cortical structures of the planum temporale by planimetry of serial sections on Nissl and myelin stained whole brain coronal sections of postmortem brains of 19 schizophrenic patients and 20 matched nonpsychiatric control subjects. The mean anterior–posterior diameter of the PT was significantly reduced in the left hemisphere (-16%, $p < .03$), but unchanged on the right side. PT asymmetry (expressed as a left/right volume ratio) was more reduced in male patients (-25%, $p < .20$) than in female schizophrenics (-2%, $p < .95$). Schizophrenic patients demonstrated an 8% volume reduction of left PT (males: -5%, ns; females: -10%, ns), whereas the right PT volume was increased in male schizophrenics only ($+14\%$, ns) but moderately decreased in female patients (-4%, ns)[108].

As already described above, we recently found a significant increase of 'abnormally positioned' pre-alpha cell groups in the left entorhinal cortex of schizophrenics by 43% ($p < .03$). There was a diagnosis by side interaction for the left ($p < .05$) but not for the right hemisphere. Patients with a family history of psychiatric illness had significantly more misplaced neurons in the left hemisphere compared to patients lacking such a history. Finally, there was a trend for more heterotopias in the left but not in the right entorhinal cortex in patients with an early onset of the disease[103].

Taken together, there is growing evidence from postmortem and MRI studies that there is increased prevalence of left hemispheric/temporal lobe pathology in schizophrenia. This is possibly the consequence of disturbed brain lateralization.

What is brain lateralization? Since Broca[109] we know that in humans each brain hemisphere has specific functions and that sensoric input does not reach each hemisphere to the same extent.

Which parts of the human brain are lateralized? The major anatomical components of hominization in the central nervous system are a gross allometric enlargement of the whole brain, selective enlargement of the parietal and frontal lobes, Broca's and Wernicke's area and development of moderate to marked asymmetry particularly of the postrolandic part of the lateral (Sylvian) fissure[110].

Is there a necessity for cerebral lateralization in human evolution? Crow speculated in a recent paper[111] that increasing social interactions and language are a likely explanation for the development of laterality in the human brain. The concept of the 'social brain'[112] attempts to account for the neural apparatus required for such interactions, in particular for the extent to which primate brain evolution has been dependent upon the development of a capacity for recognizing and communicating with conspecifics. The 'social brain' includes mechanisms for identifying others, eg through the recognition of specific facial features, as a mean of ascertaining their 'intentions' towards oneself. The areas of the brain which are envisaged as being particularly relevant include the region of the superior temporal sulcus, the amygdala and the orbital frontal cortex.

What do we know about the mechanisms of histological asymmetry in the human brain? From experimental data in the rat brain we know that histological asymmetry is a result of changes in cell numbers and not cell packing density. It is assumed that, in both hemispheres, the same amount of neurons migrate to their final destination. Asymmetry is a consequence of later occurring regressive events especially programmed cell death[113]. Interhemispheric connections differ between symmetrical and asymmetrical brain regions. As volumetric asymmetry increases, the percentage of axonal termination decreases, partly as a result of a decrease in the number of patches of callosal axonal termination[114]. The latter finding is supported by the fact that the corpus callosum in left handers is thicker than in right handed people[115]. The planum temporale asymmetry is lost in most left handed people, whereas, in right handed people, the left planum is two to three times thicker than the right one[107].

Is there disturbed laterality in psychiatric disorders? Since the fine work of Geschwind and Levitzky[116] on planum temporale asymmetries in the human brain, cerebral asymmetries received increased attention in research. Today, we know that, in healthy right handed people, usually the left Sylvian fissure, the left planum temporale, the right frontal lobe and the left occipital lobe are bigger than their contralateral partners. These asymmetries are largely present at birth and develop genetically preprogrammed in the second and third trimester of pregnancy[117–119]. There is now some evidence that this anatomical cerebral asymmetry is reduced, absent, or reversed in persons with left handedness[107], dyslexia[120] and autism[121]. Schizophrenia might be another candidate in this list, and it is interesting to note that, as early as 1969, Flor-Henry reported an increased frequency of schizophrenia-like psychosis in temporal lobe epileptics with a left hemispheric focus, while right hemispheric fits were associated with affective disorders[122]. There are, however, many more neurophysiological[123,124] and biochemical[125] studies indicating that the left brain hemisphere is deficient in schizophrenia. Looking at our recent postmortem data on the planum temporale cortical volumes, we found a *decrease* of the volume on the left side and an *increase* on the right side at least in male schizophrenia. That indicates that the planum temporale cortical volume is not only reduced in the left hemisphere but the *pattern of asymmetry* of this structure is *disrupted in schizophrenia*. The absolute amount of changes is small (left: 5%, right: +14%), but the effects of them might be disastrous for the rest of brain as indicated in a recent study. In an attempt to determine the true magnitude of cellular and fibre disruption associated with the presence of ectopias, cortical sections from autoimmune mice containing ectopias were stained for a specific neurofilament. Ectopias are subpially misplaced neurons, a circumscribed indicator for a disturbance of late neuronal migration. The neurofilament stained sections revealed substantial disruption of the cortical layers underlying the ectopic neurons. This resulted primarily from the existence of dense, radially oriented fibre bundles spanning the thickness of the cortex underlying the ectopias. In some instances, these fibre bundles could be seen to join the corpus callosum[126].

Summary and conclusions

The pathomorphological changes in schizophrenia are subtle and not comparable in magnitude to the brain tissue loss seen in the well known degenerative brain disorders. The changes cannot be seen in all schizophrenic patients. There is a considerable overlap between patients and healthy controls and, morphometrically, only a minority (some 20–30%) have values below the range of matched healthy control cases. Recent MRI studies examining different areas of the brain of schizophrenic patients suggest that the major locus of pathology is the temporal lobe with the hippocampus, amygdala and entorhinal cortex[37–40,42–45,127].

Lack of gliosis and lack of a positive correlation with length of illness are arguments as least in most patients for the fact that the structural changes are not progressive and were probably acquired very early in life[24,105,128–132].

Since both hemispheres are examined in postmortem studies, the evidence shows that there is an increased prevalence of lesions in the left hemisphere, specifically in the left temporal lobe in schizophrenia. One possible explanation is damage to the brain at a time when the right hemisphere is mature but the left hemisphere is still growing and therefore more vulnerable. Another explanation could be a disturbance of brain lateralization in general. This would, for instance, account for the decrease of planum temporale cortical volume on the left side but an increase on the right side in male schizophrenia[108]. It would lead only to subtle volume differences but to a general miswiring of the brain. Depending on the extent of wrongly placed connections, the brain will function for some time, because not all connections are activated before puberty. Under the influence of additional factors related to the vulnerable age period between puberty and old age, such as late myelination in the frontal or limbic cortex[128,133], steroid hormones[129], abnormal synaptic sprouting[134], or psychosocial stressors[135], these wrongly placed wires will become active enabling a person to become psychotic. We hypothesize that, in most schizophrenic patients, cerebral laterality is disturbed. Depending on the degree of disturbance, negative symptoms will prevail, while patients with nearly undisturbed laterality, but limbic pathology, will have mainly positive symptoms[136].

Acknowledgement

This work was supported by the Deutsche Forschungsgemeinschaft (Bo 799/1–3) and the Krupp-von Bohlen und Halbach Stiftung.

References

(1) Alzheimer A. Beiträge zur pathologischen Anatomie der Hirnrinde und zur anatomischen Grundlage der Psychosen. *Mschr Psychiat Neurol* 1897; 2: 82–120.
(2) Stevens JR. An anatomy of schizophrenia? *Arch Gen Psychiat* 1973; 29: 177–89.
(3) David GB. The pathological anatomy of the schizophrenias. In: Richter D, ed. *Schizophrenia: somatic aspects*. Oxford: Pergamon Press, 1957: 93–130.
(4) Jellinger K. Neuromorphological background of pathochemical studies in major psychoses. In: Beckmann H, Riederer P eds. *Pathochemical markers in major psychoses*. Heidelberg: Springer, 1985: 1–23.
(5) Kirch D, Weinberger DR. Anatomical neuropathology in schizophrenia: postmortem findings. In: Nasrallah HA, Weinberger DR, eds. *The neurology of schizophrenia*. New York: Elsevier, 1986: 325–48.
(6) Broser K. Hirngewicht und Hirnprozeß bei Schizophrenie. *Arch Psychiat Nervenkr* 1949; 182: 439–49.
(7) Jellinger K. Zur Neuropathologie schizophrener Psychosen. *Curr Top Neuropathol* 1980; 6: 85–99.
(8) Brown R, Colter N, Corsellis JAN et al. Postmortem evidence of structural brain changes in schizophrenia. Differences in brain weight, temporal horn area and parahippocampal gyrus compared with affective disorder. *Arch Gen Psychiat* 1986; 43: 36–42.
(9) Pakkenberg B. Post-mortem study of chronic schizophrenic brains. *Br J Psychiat* 1987; 151: 744–52.
(10) Bruton CJ, Crow TJ, Frith CD, Johnstone EC, Owens DGC, Roberts GW. Schizophrenia and the brain: a prospective clinico-neuropathological study. *Psych Med* 1990; 20: 285–304.
(11) Heckers S, Heinsen H, Geiger B, Beckmann H. Hippocampal neuron number in schizophrenia. *Arch Gen Psychiat* 1991b; 48: 1002–8.
(12) Bogerts B, Meertz E, Schönfeldt-Bausch R. Limbic system pathology in schizophrenia: a controlled post-mortem study. VII. *World Congress of Psychiatry*, Wien, 1983b: Vortrag, Abst F6.

P Falkai and B Bogerts

(13) Bogerts B. Zur Neuropathologie der Schizophrenien. *Fortschr Neurol Psychiat* 1984; 52: 428–37.
(14) Bogerts B. Schizophrenien als Erkrankungen des limbischen Systems. In: Huber G ed. *Basisstadien endogener Psychosen und das Borderline-Problem.* Stuttgart: Schattauer, 1985: 163–79.
(15) Bogerts B, David S, Falkai P, Tapernon-Franz U. Quantitative evaluation of astrocyte densities in schizophrenia. Presented at the *17th Congress of the Collegium Internationale Neuro-Psychopharmacologicum*, Kyoto, 1990c: Abst P-13-1-22.
(16) Kovelmann JA, Scheibel AB. A neurohistological correlate of schizophrenia. *Biol Psychiat* 1984; 19: 1601–21.
(17) Jakob J, Beckmann H. Prenatal developmental disturbances in the limbic allocortex in schizophrenics. *J Neural Transm* 1986; 65: 303–26.
(18) Falkai P, Bogerts B. Cell loss in the hippocampus of schizophrenics. *Eur Arch Psychiat Neurol Sci* 1986; 236: 154–61.
(19) Falkai P, Bogerts B. Morphometric evidence for developmental disturbances in brains of some schizophrenics. *Schizophr Res* 1989; 2(1–2): 99.
(20) Falkai P, Bogerts B, Rozumek M. Cell loss and volume reduction in the entorhinal cortex of schizophrenics. *Biol Psychiat* 1988a; 24: 515–21.
(21) Falkai P, Bogerts B, Greve B, Schneider Th, Pfeiffer U, Machus B. A semiquantitative assessment of heterotopic pre-alpha-cell clusters in the entorhinal cortex of schizophrenic patients. *Br J Psychiat* 1992b; (submitted).
(22) Colter N, Battal S, Crow TJ, Johnstone EC, Brown R, Bruton Cl. White matter reduction in the parahippocampal gyrus of patients with schizophrenia. *Arch Gen Psychiat* 1987; 44: 1023.
(23) Jeste DV, Lohr JB. Hippocampal pathologic findings in schizophrenia. A morphometric study. *Arch Gen Psychiat* 1989; 46: 1019–24.
(24) Crow TJ, Ball J, Bloom StR et al. Schizophrenia as an anomaly of development of cerebral asymmetry. *Arch Gen Psychiat* 1989; 46: 1145–50.
(25) Altshuler LL, Casanova MP, Goldberg TE, Kleinman JE. The hippocampus and parahippocampus in schizophrenic, suicide, and control brains. *Arch Gen Psychiat* 1990; 47: 1029–34.
(26) Casanova MF, Saunder R, Altshuler L et al. Entorhinal cortex pathology in schizophrenia and affective disorders. In: Racagni G et al. eds. *Biological psychiatry*, Amsterdam: Elsevier, 1991c; 504–6.
(27) Benes FM, Bird ED. An analysis of the arrangement of neurons in the cingulate cortex of schizophrenic patients. *Arch Gen Psychiat* 1987; 44: 608–16.
(28) Benes FM, Majocha R, Bird ED, Marotta CA. Increased vertical axon numbers in cingulate cortex of schizophrenics. *Arch Gen Psychiat* 1987; 44: 1017–21.
(29) Benes FM, McSparren J, Bird ED, SanGiovanni JP, Vincent SL. Deficits in small interneurons in prefrontal and cingulate cortices of schizophrenic and schizoaffective patients. *Arch Gen Psychiat* 1991a; 48: 996–1001.
(30) Benes FM, Sorensen I, Bird ED. Reduced neuronal size in posterior hippocampus of schizophrenic patients. *Schizophrenia Bull* 1991b; 17(4): 597–608.
(31) Arnold SE, Hyman BT, VanHösen GW, Damasio AR. Some cytoarchitectural abnormalities of the entorhinal cortex in schizophrenia. *Arch Gen Psychiat* 1991; 48: 625–32.

(32) Conrad AJ, Abebe T, Austin R, Forsythe S, Scheibel AB. Hippocampal cell disarray in schizophrenia. *Arch Gen Psychiat* 1991; 48: 413–17.

(33) Heckers S, Heinsen H, Heinsen Y, Beckmann H. Cortex, white matter, and basal ganglia in schizophrenia: a volumetric postmortem study. 1991a; 29: 556–66.

(34) Christison GW, Casanova MF, Weinberger DR, Rawlings R, Kleinman JE. A quantitative investigation of hippocampal pyramidal cell size, shape and variability of orientation in schizophrenia. *Arch Gen Psychiat* 1989; 46: 1027–32.

(35) Heckers S, Heinsen H, Heinsen Y, Beckmann H. Morphometry of the parahippocampal gyrus in schizophrenics and controls. Some anatomical considerations. *J Neural Transm* 1990a; 80: 151–5.

(36) Heckers S, Heinsen H, Heinsen YC, Beckmann H. Limbic structures and lateral ventricle in schizophrenia. *Arch Gen Psychiat* 1990b; 47: 1016–22.

(37) DeLisi LE, Dauphinais ID, Gershon E. Perinatal complications and reduced size of brain limbic structures in familial schizophrenia. *Schizophrenia Bull* 1988; 14: 185–91.

(38) Suddath RL, Casanova MF, Goldberg TE, Daniel DG, Kelsoe J, Weinberger DR. Temporal lobe pathology in schizophrenia: a quantitative magnetic resonance imaging study. *Am J Psychiat* 1989; 146: 464–72.

(39) Suddath RL, Christison GW, Torrey EF, Casanova MF, Weinberger DR. Anatomical abnormalities in the brains of monozygotic twins discordant for schizophrenia. *New Eng J Med* 1990; 322(12): 62–7.

(40) Rossi A, Stratta P, D'Albenzio L et al. Reduced temporal lobe areas in schizophrenia: preliminary evidences from a controlled multiplanar magnetic resonance imaging study. *Biol Psychiat* 1990; 27: 61–8.

(41) Bogerts B, Falkai P, Haupts M et al. Post-mortem volume measurements of limbic system and basal ganglia structures in chronic schizophrenics. *Schizophr Res* 1990b; 3: 295–301.

(42) Becker T, Elmer K, Mechela B et al. MRI findings in medial temporal lobe structures in schizophrenia. *Europ Neuropsychopharmacol* 1990; 1: 83–6.

(43) Barta PE, Pearlson GD, Powers RE, Richards SS, Tune LE. Reduced volume of superior temporal gyrus in schizophrenia: relationship to auditory hallucinations. *Am J Psychiat* 1990; 147: 1457–62.

(44) Dauphinais D, DeLisi LE, Crow TJ et al. Reduction in temporal lobe size in siblings with schizophrenia: a magnetic resonance imaging study. *Psychiat Res* 1990; 35: 137–47.

(45) Jernigan TL, Zisook S, Heaton RK, Moranville JT, Hesselink JR, Braff DL. Magnetic resonance imaging abnormalities in lenticular nuclei and cerebral cortex in schizophrenia. *Arch Gen Psychiat* 1991; 48: 881–90.

(46) Casanova M, Atkinson D, Goldberg T et al. A quantitative morphometric study of the corpus callosum and cingulate cortex in schizophrenia. In: Racagni G et al. eds. *Biological psychiatry*. Amsterdam: Elsevier, 1991a: 373–5.

(47) Degreef G, Bogerts B, Falkai P et al. Increased prevalence of the cavum septum pellucidum in MRI scans and postmortem brains of schizophrenic patients. *Psychiat Res: Neuroimag* 1992; 45: 1–13.

(48) Southard EE. On the topographic distribution of cortex lesions and anomalies

in dementia praecox with some account of their functional significance. *Am J Insanity* 1915; 71: 603–71.

(49) Colon EJ. Quantitative cytoarchitectonics of the human cerebral cortex in schizophrenic dementia. *Acta Neuropathol*, Berl, 1972; 20: 1–10.

(50) Benes FM, Davidson B, Bird ED. Quantitative cytoarchitectural studies of the cerebral cortex of schizophrenics. *Arch Gen Psychiat* 1986; 43: 31–5.

(51) Rosenthal R, Bigelow LB. Quantitative brain measurements in chronic schizophrenia. *Br J Psychiat* 1972; 121: 259–64.

(52) Bogerts B, Ashtari M, Degreef G, Alvir JMaJ, Bilder RM, Lieberman JA. Reduced temporal limbic structure volumes on magnetic resonance images in first episode schizophrenia. *Psychiat Res: Neuroimag* 1990a; 35: 1–13.

(53) Stevens JR. Clinicopathological correlations in schizophrenia. *Arch Gen Psychiat* 1986; 43: 715–16.

(54) Dom R, de Saedeler J, Bogerts B, Hopf A. Quantitative cytometric analysis of basal ganglia in catatonic schizophrenics. In: Perris et al. eds. *Biological psychiatry*, Amsterdam: Elsevier, 723–6.

(55) Swayze VW, Andreasen NC, Alliger RJ, Yuh WTC, Ehrhard JC. Subcortical and temporal structures in affective disorders and schizophrenia: a magnetic resonance imaging study. *Biol Psychiat* 1992; 31: 221–40.

(56) Hopf A. Orientierende Untersuchung zur Frage pathoanatomischer Veränderungen im Pallidum und Striatum bei Schizophrenie. *J Hirnforsch* 1954; 1: 97–145.

(57) Stevens JR. Neuropathology of schizophrenia. *Arch Gen Psychiat* 1982; 39: 1131–9.

(58) Bogerts B, Meertz E, Schönfeld-Bausch R. Basal ganglia and limbic system pathology in schizophrenia. *Arch Gen Psychiat* 1985; 42: 784–91.

(59) Early TS, Reiman EM, Raichle ME et al. Left globus pallidus abnormality in never-medicated patients with schizophrenia. *Proc Nat Acad Sci USA* 1987; 84: 561–3.

(60) Luchins DL, Metz JT, Marks RC, Cooper MD. Basal ganglia glucose metabolism asymmetry during a catatonic episode. *Biol Psychiat* 1989; 26: 725–8.

(61) Mesulam MM. Patterns in behavioral neuroanatomy: association areas, the limbic system, and hemispheric specialization. In: Mesulam MM ed. *Principles of behavioral neurology*. Philadelphia: Davis, 1986: 1–70.

(62) Nasrallah HA, Andreasen NC, Coffman JA et al. A controlled magnetic resonance imaging study of corpus callosum thickness in schizophrenia. *Biol Psychiat* 1986; 21: 274–82.

(63) Raine A, Harrison GN, Reynolds GP, Sheard Ch, Cooper JE, Medley I. Structural and functional characteristics of the corpus callosum in schizophrenics, psychiatric controls and normal controls. *Arch Gen Psychiat* 1990; 47: 1060–4.

(64) Mathew PJ, Partain CL. Midsagittal sections of the cerebellar vermis and fourth ventricle obtained with magnetic resonance imaging in schizophrenic patients. *Am J Psychiat* 1985; 142(8): 970–1.

(65) Uematso M, Kaiya H. The morphology of the corpus callosum in schizophrenia: an MRI study. *Schizophr Res* 1988; 1: 391–8.

(66) Rossi A, Stratta P, Gallucci M, Passarellio R, Cassachia M. Quantification of

corpus callosum and ventricles in schizophrenia with nuclear magnetic resonance imaging: a pilot study. *Am J Psychiat* 1989; 146: 99–101.

(67) Bogerts B, Lesch A, Lange H, Zech M, Tutsch J. Hypotrophy of the corpus callosum in schizophrenia. *Neurosci Lett* 1983c; (suppl) 34.

(68) Günther W, Moser E, Petsch R, Brodie JD, Steinberg R, Streck P. Pathological cerebral blood flow and corpus callosum abnormalities in schizophrenia: relations to EEG mapping and Pet data. *Psychiat Res* 1989; 29: 453–5.

(69) Fünfgeld E. Pathologisch-anatomische Untersuchungen bei Dementia praecox mit besonderer Berücksichtigung des Thalamus opticus. *Z Ges Neurol Psychiat* 1925; 95: 411–63.

(70) Bäumer H. Veränderungen des Thalamus bei Schizophrenie. *J Hirnforsch* 1954; 1: 157–72.

(71) Treff WM, Hempel KJ. Die Zelldichte bei Schizophrenen und klinisch Gesunden. *J Hirnforsch* 1958; 4: 314–69.

(72) Lesch A, Bogerts B. The diencephalon in schizophrenia: evidence for reduced thickness of the periventricular grey matter. *Eur Arch Psychiat Neurol Sci* 1984; 234: 212–9.

(73) Pakkenberg B. Pronounced reduction of total neuron number in mediodorsal thalamic nucleus and nucleus accumbens in schizophrenics. *Arch Gen Psychiat* 1990; 47: 1023–8.

(74) Huber G. Die coenaesthetische Schizophrenie. *Fortschr Neurol Psychiat* 1957; 25: 491–520.

(75) Gross G, Huber G. Sensorische Störungen bei Schizophrenien. *Arch Psychiat Nervenkr* 1972; 216: 119–30.

(76) Gross G, Huber G, Schüttler R. Computerized tomography studies on schizophrenic diseases. *Arch Psychiat Nervenkr* 1982; 231: 519–26.

(77) Averback P. Lesions of the nucleus ansae peduncularis in neuropsychiatric disease. *Arch Neurol* 1981a; 38: 230–5.

(78) Arendt T, Bigl Y, Arendt A, Tennstedt A. Loss of neurons in the nucleus basalis of Meynert in Alzheimer's disease, paralysis agitans and Korsakoff's disease. *Acta Neuropathol*, Berl 1983; 61: 101–8.

(79) Lohr JB, Jeste DV. Locus ceruleus morphometry in aging and schizophrenia. *Acta Psychiat Scand* 1988; 77: 689–97.

(80) Karson CN, Garcia-Rill E, Biedermann JA, Mrak RE, Husain MM, Skinner RD. The brain stem reticular formation in schizophrenia. *Pyschiat Res: Neuroimag* 1991; 40: 31–48.

(81) Duchen LW. General pathology of neurons and neuroglia. In: Adams JH, Corsellis JAN, Duchen LW, eds. *Greenfield's neuropathology* 4th edn. London: Edward Arnold, 1984: 27–45.

(82) Rakic P. Mode of cell migration to the superficial layers of fetal monkey neocortex. *J Comp Neurol* 1972; 145: 61–84.

(83) Rakic P. Specification of cerebral cortical areas. *Science* 1988; 241: 170–6.

(84) Peters A, Palay SL, Webster H deF. *The fine structure of the nervous system*, 2nd edn. Philadelphia: Saunders, 1976.

(85) Hertz L. An intense potassium uptake into astrocytes, its further enhancement by high concentrations of potassium and its possible involvement in potassium homeostasis at the cellular level. *Brain Res* 1978; 145: 202–8.

(86) Hertz L. Drug-induced alterations of ion distribution at the cellular level of the central nervous system. *Pharmacol Rev* 1977; 26: 250–8.

(87) Friede RL. *Developmental neuropathology.* Berlin: Springer-Verlag, 1989.

(88) Polak M, Haymaker W, Johnson JE, D'Amelio F, Hager H. Neuroglia and their reaction. In: Haymaker W, Adams RD, eds. *Histology and histopathology of the nervous system*, vol.I, New Springfield, IL: Charles C Thomas, 1982: Chap 5, pp. 363–480.

(89) Fisman M. The brain stem in psychosis. *Br J Psychiat* 1975; 126: 414–22.

(90) Nieto D, Escobar A. Major psychoses. In: Minkler J, ed. *Pathology of the nervous system.* New York: McGraw-Hill, 1972; 2654–65.

(91) Roberts GW, Colter N, Lofthouse R, Bogerts B, Zech M, Crow TJ. Gliosis in schizophrenia: a survey. *Biol Psychiat* 1986; 21: 1043–50.

(92) Roberts GW, Colter N, Lofthouse R, Johnstone EC, Crow TJ. Is there gliosis in schizophrenia? Investigations of the temporal lobe. *Biol Psychiat* 1987; 22: 1459–68.

(93) Stevens CD, Altshuler LL, Bogerts B, Falkai P. Quantitative study of gliosis in schizophrenia and Huntington's chorea. *Biol Psychiat* 1988; 24: 697–700.

(94) Bogerts B, Häntsch H, Herzer M. A morphometric study of the dopamine-containing cell groups in the mesencephalon of normals, Parkinson patients and schizophrenics. *Biol Psychiat* 1983a; 18: 951–71.

(95) Casanova MF, Stevens JR, Kleinman JE. Quantitation of astrocytes in the molecular layer of the dentate gyrus: a study in schizophrenia and Alzheimer's disease patients. *Psychiat Res* 1991b; in press.

(96) Woods BT, Yurgelun Todd D, Benes FM, Frankenburg FR, Pope HG, McSparren J. Progressive ventricular enlargement in schizophrenia: comparison to bipolar disorder and correlation with clinical course. *Biol Psychiat* 1990; 27: 341–52.

(97) Bayer SA, Altman J. *Neocortical development.* New York: Raven Press, 1991: Chap 1, 3–10.

(98) Caviness VS. Normal development of cerebral neocortex. In: Evrard P, Minkowski A, eds. *Developmental neurobiology.* Nestlé Nutrition Workshop Series, vol. 12, New York: Vevey/Raven Press Ltd, 1989: 1–10.

(99) McLardy T. Hippocampal zinc and structural deficit in brains from chronic alcoholics and some schizophrenics. *J Orthomol Psychiat* 1974; 4(1): 32–6.

(100) Scheibel AB, Kovelman JA. Disorientation of the hippocampal pyramidal cells and its processes in the schizophrenic patient. *Biol Psychiat* 1981; 16: 101–2.

(101) Altshuler L, Conrad A, Kovelman JA, Scheibel A. Hippocampal pyramidal cell orientation in schizophrenia. *Arch Gen Psychiat* 1987; 44: 1094–8.

(102) Jakob H, Beckmann H. Gross and histological criteria for developmental disorders in brains of schizophrenics. *J Roy Soc Med* 1989; 82(8): 466–9.

(103) Falkai P, Bogerts B, Greve B et al. Loss of Sylvian fissure asymmetry in schizophrenia. A quantitative postmortem study. *Schizophr Res* 1992; 7: 23–32.

(104) Friede RL. *Developmental neuropathology.* Berlin: Springer-Verlag, 1975.

(105) Bogerts B. The neuropathology of schizophrenia. In: Häfner H, Gattaz WF, eds. *Search for the causes of schizophrenia.* Berlin: Springer-Verlag, 1990: 229–241.

(106) Crow TJ, Brown R, Bruton CJ, Frith CD, Gray V. Loss of Sylvian fissure asymmetry in schizophrenia: findings in the Runwell 2 series of brains. *Schizophr Res* 1992; 6(2): 152–3.
(107) Steinmetz H, Volkmann J, Jäncke J, Freund HJ. Anatomical left–right asymmetry of language-related temporal cortex is different in left- and right-handers. *Ann Neurol* 1991; 29: 315–9.
(108) Falkai P, Bogerts B, Greve B et al. Reduced Sylvian fissure and planum temporale asymmetry in schizophrenia. Evidence for disturbed left hemispheric neurodevelopment? *Schizophr Res* 1992c; 6(2): 152.
(109) Broca P. 1864 cited from: Critchley M: *Aphasiology and other aspects of language.* London: Arnold, 1970.
(110) Tobias PV. The anatomy of hominization. In: Vidrio EA, Galina MA, eds. *Advances in the morphology of cells and tissues.* New York: Alan R Liss, 1981: 101–10.
(111) Crow TJ. The origins of psychosis and 'The descent of man'. *Br J Psychiat* 1991; 159(14): 76–82.
(112) Brothers L. The social brain: a project for integrating primate behavior and neurophysiology in a new domain. *Concepts in Neurosci* 1990; 15: 27–51.
(113) Galaburda AM, Aboitiz F, Rosen GD, Sherman GF. Histological asymmetry in the primary visual cortex of the rat: implications for mechanisms of cerebral asymmetry. *Cortex* 1986; 22: 151–60.
(114) Rosen GD, Sherman FG, Galaburda AM. Interhemispheric connections differ between symmetrical and asymmetrical brain regions. *Neurosci* 1989; 33(3): 525–33.
(115) Witelson SF. Hand preference and sex differences in the isthmus of the corpus callosum. *Soc Neurosci* Abstr, 1987; 13, 48.
(116) Geschwind N, Levitsky. Human brain: Left–right asymmetries in temporal speech region. *Science* 1968; 161: 186–7.
(117) Witelson SF, Pallie W. Left hemisphere specialisation for language in the newborn: neuroanatomical evidence of asymmetry. *Brain* 1973; 96: 641–7.
(118) Wada JA, Clarke R, Hamm A. Cerebral hemispheric asymmetries in humans. *Arch Neurol* 1975; 32: 239–46.
(119) Wada JA, Davies AE. Fundamental nature of human infant's brain asymmetry. *Can J Neurol Sci* 1977; 4: 203–7.
(120) Galaburda AM, Habib M. Cerebral dominance: biological associations and pathology. *Discuss Neurosci* 1987; IV. Geneva: Foundation FESN.
(121) Prior MR, Bradshaw JL. Hemispheric functioning in autistic children. *Cortex* 1979; 15: 73–81.
(122) Flor-Henry P. Psychosis and temporal lobe epilepsy: a controlled investigation. *Epilepsia* 1969; 10: 363–95.
(123) Gruzelier J, Hammond N. Schizophrenia – a dominant hemisphere temporal lobe disorder? *Res Commun Psych, Psychiat Behav* 1976; 1: 33–72.
(124) Schweitzer L, Becker E, Welsh H. Abnormalities of cerebral lateralisation in schizophrenic patients. *Arch Gen Psychiat* 1978; 35: 982–5.
(125) Reynolds GP. Increased concentrations and lateral asymmetry of amygdala dopamine in schizophrenia. *Nature* 1983; 305: 527–9.
(126) Sherman GF, Stone JS, Press DM, Rosen GD, Galaburda AM. Abnormal

architecture and connections disclosed by neurofilament staining in the cerebral cortex of autoimmune mice. *Brain Res* 1990; 529: 202-7.

(127) Young AH, Blackwood DHR, Roxborough H, McQueen JK, Martin MJ, Kean D. A magnetic resonance imaging study of schizophrenia: brain structure and clinical symptoms. *Br J Psychiat* 1991; 158: 158-64.

(128) Weinberger DR. Implications of normal brain development for the pathogenesis of schizophrenia. *Arch Gen Psychiat* 1987; 44: 660-9.

(129) Bogerts B. Limbic and paralimbic pathology in schizophrenia: interaction with age and stress related factors. In: Schulz SC, Tamminga CA, eds. *Schizophrenia: scientific progress.* Oxford: Oxford University Press, 1989; 216-27.

(130) Bogerts B. The neuropathology of schizophrenia: pathophysiological and neurodevelopmental implications. In: Mednick SA, Cannon TD, Barr CE, eds. *Fetal neural development and adult schizophrenia.* Cambridge: Cambridge University Press, 1991: 153-73.

(131) Roberts GW. Schizophrenia: a neuropathological perspective. *Br J Psychiat* 1991; 158: 8-17.

(132) Jones P, Murray RM. The genetics of schizophrenia is the genetics of neurodevelopment. *Br J Psychiat* 1991; 158: 615-23.

(133) Benes FM. Myelination of cortical-hippocampal relays during late adolescence. *Schizophr Bull* 1989; 15: 585-93.

(134) Stevens JR. Schizophrenia: static or progressive pathophysiology? *Schizophr Res* 1991; 5: 184-6.

(135) Zubin J, Spring B. Vulnerability – a new view of schizophrenia. *J Abnorm Psycho* 1977; 86: 103-26.

(136) Bilder RM, Degreef G. Morphological markers of neurodevelopmental paths to schizophrenia. In: Mednick SA, Cannon TD, Barr CE, Lafosse JM, eds. *Developmental pathology of schizophrenia.* New York: Plenum, 1992: 167-90.

(137) Bigelow LB, Nasrallah HA, Rauscher FP. Corpus callosum thickness in chronic schizophrenia. *Br J Psychiat* 1983; 142: 282-7.

(138) Nasrallah HA, McCalley-Whitters M, Rauscher FP et al. A histological study of the corpus callosum in chronic schizophrenia. *Psych Res* 1983; 8: 151-60.

(139) Bogerts B, Falkai P, Tutsch J. Cell numbers in the pallidum and hippocampus of schizophrenics. In: Shagass C et al. eds. *Biological psychiatry.* Amsterdam: Elsevier, 1986: 1178-80.

Neuroendocrine developments in psychiatric research

J A BEARN and P W RAVEN

Introduction

Many of the early neuroendocrine studies in psychiatric disorder were purely descriptive, relying on relatively simple techniques such as plasma hormone measurement. In part, this is an inevitable stage, which any new field has to go through, in order to identify more closely those psychiatric disorders in which further and more detailed study of endocrine mechanisms is merited. As a consequence, many psychiatrists still see neuroendocrine abnormalities in psychiatric disorder as epiphenomena.

In fact, the development of new techniques and growth in our understanding of neuroendocrine physiology have allowed 3 main lines of research to develop: first, studies aimed at improving the depth of our knowledge about those areas where the association between psychiatric disorder and endocrine abnormality is the strongest; secondly, studies utilizing neuroendocrine probes to gain information regarding the functioning of neurotransmitter systems in vivo; and thirdly, the roles of hormones in neurodevelopment and cognitive function.

We will discuss recent developments in each of these areas of research, focusing on major depressive illness as this is the disorder which has been most extensively studied from the neuroendocrine perspective, and in which the findings are most robust. Our intention is to demonstrate that, as in other areas of psychiatric research, neuroendocrine studies have now moved on from the purely descriptive to the explanatory model, and are now aimed at increasing our understanding of how neuroendocrine mechanisms contribute to the pathophysiology of psychiatric disorder with a view to developing rational treatment strategies.

All correspondence to: Dr J A Bearn, Section of Sciences of Addiction, Institute of Psychiatry, De Crespigny Park, London SE5 8AF, UK

Cambridge Medical Reviews: Neurobiology and Psychiatry Volume 2
© Cambridge University Press

The hypothalamo-pituitary-adrenal axis in affective disorders

The hypothalamo-pituitary-adrenal (HPA) axis plays a crucial, but paradoxical, role in the adaptive response to stress: increased HPA activity both potentiates the protective catabolic response to acute stress and acts to damp down the primary stress response, thus restoring homeostasis. Failure to either mount or terminate the HPA stress response appropriately leads to maladaptation and disease. There is growing evidence that one of the protective functions of the HPA axis may be considered the homeostasis of euthymia, through the effects of its hormones on neurochemical systems which contribute to mood and behaviour[1].

In the healthy individual perception of stress results in hypothalamic release of corticotropin-releasing hormone (CRH) and other corticotropin (ACTH) secretagogues, especially vasopressin (AVP). These factors stimulate the anterior pituitary to release ACTH, which, in turn stimulates the adrenal cortex to secrete corticosteroids, notably the glucocorticoid, cortisol. In the absence of continuing stress the HPA response is terminated via a closed loop feedback system whereby glucocorticoids act on the pituitary, hypothalamus and hippocampus to decrease further release of CRH and ACTH[2].

In 50–60% of patients with major depressive disorder there are measurable abnormalities of the HPA axis, including hypersecretion of CRH and cortisol, altered cortisol Circadian rhythm, resistance to suppression of cortisol by the synthetic glucocorticoid dexamethasone and adrenal gland hypertrophy[3,4]. The currently favoured explanation for this maladaptive stress response in affective disorders is that 'limbic system–hypothalamic overdrive of CRH' results in dysregulation at several sites in the HPA axis[5]. This concept derives equally from predominantly animal studies of hippocampal corticosteroid receptors and dynamic tests utilizing CRH in the human.

Hippocampal corticosteroid receptors

There are two different cytosolic receptors for corticosteroids[6]. The type I or mineralocorticoid receptor (MR) has high affinity for aldosterone and the glucocorticoids cortisol and corticosterone, but lower affinity for the synthetic steroid dexamethasone. The type II or glucocorticoid receptor (GR) has high affinity for dexamethasone, lower affinity for glucocorticoids, and much lower affinity for aldosterone. Considerable impetus has been provided to the study of the distribution and function of corticosteroid receptors in brain by the recent isolation, cloning and sequencing of cDNAs encoding both human and rat GR[7,8] and MR[9,10]. In the brain, MR are located predominantly in the hippocampus, while GR are more widely distributed, but are concentrated in the septo-hippocampal region[11]. The presence of high concentrations of both receptor subtypes in the hippocampus, recently confirmed in the human postmortem brain[12], confers considerable sensitivity of this structure to prevailing glucocorticoid levels. Tonic effects may be mediated through the low capacity MR sites which have high rates of occupancy under basal condition, while the response to stress may be mediated through the high capacity GR sites which show low occupancy under basal conditions[13].

There is considerable evidence that hippocampal corticosteroid receptors have a role in the negative feedback control of CRH secretion and, especially, in the termination of the stress response. Lesions of the hippocampus generally tend to increase HPA activity, especially after stress[14], and also affect levels of CRH and vasopressin mRNAs in the hypothalamus[15] Hippocampal lesions also produce resistance to the inhibitory effect of dexamethasone in rats[16]. The conventional view, derived from in vitro studies, held that the most important sites for glucocorticoid negative feedback are at the level of the pituitary and hypothalamus. Recent studies, however, show that corticosteroid receptors in the hippocampus are more sensitive than those in the pituitary or hypothalamus to variations in circulating levels of endogenous glucocorticoids as measured by receptor activation[13] or receptor mRNA levels[17]. Overall, the hippocampus appears to have a significant role in the fast-feedback control of the HPA[2,15].

Glucocorticoids, acting through hippocampal receptors, have additional effects which may be relevant in affective disorders. Within the hippocampus they influence serotonin (5HT) turnover and 5HT receptor capacity[18], binding at $5HT_{1A}$ and $5HT_{1B}$ receptors[19], the electrophysiological response to serotonin and other monoamines[20], GABA uptake[21] and β-adrenergic receptor binding[22]. In addition, the hippocampus is an area known to be associated with memory and learning, and also plays a role in the diurnal variation of glucocorticoid secretion and the anticipation of events that depend on the time of the day, such as eating[1].

Animal studies have shown that chronic stress and exposure to high levels of glucocorticoids results in down regulation of hippocampal corticosteroid receptors, leading Sapolsky et al. to suggest this as the mechanism of resistance to the dexamethasone suppression test in depressive disorder[2]. Overexposure to glucocorticoids can result in hippocampal neuronal damage, probably mediated via excitatory amino acids[23], resulting in disinhibition of the HPA and a further increase in corticosteroid levels. This glucocorticoid cascade hypothesis[2] has been suggested as a possible mechanism in the disinhibition of the HPA in depression[23]. In addition, hippocampal corticosteroid receptor expression is regulated by other hormones, eg ACTH[24] and thyroxine[25], and also by serotonergic neural activity[26]. There thus exists a theoretical framework wherein hippocampal corticosteroid receptors, with roles in the modulation of HPA and neural activity, and sensitive to neuroendocrine and monoaminergic regulation, could also have a significant role in the increased HPA activity seen in affective disorder.

In the rat, it has been shown that down-regulation of peripheral blood leukocyte GR mirrors that of hippocampal GR, although hippocampal GR are more sensitive to this process[27]. This has led to the suggestion that peripheral leukocytes in the human may serve as readily available markers reflecting changes in corticosteroid receptor levels in the brain. Most studies of lymphocyte GR in depressed patients show that levels are reduced relative to healthy controls[28,29], suggesting that down-regulation of hippocampal GR and consequent disinhibition of CRH may have a role in the HPA overactivity of depression. However, not all studies have been in agreement[30], and, in general, lymphocyte receptor studies have been performed on small groups of patients without due regard to HPA axis status, concurrent medication or time of day. The current availability of both monoclonal antibodies to the corticosteroid receptor and cDNA probes for receptor mRNA, together with our increased understanding of the effects of antidepressant treatment on corticosteroid receptors (see below), may allow useful future studies using the lymphocyte model.

CRH and dynamic tests of HPA function in affective disorders

It is increasingly recognized that CRH acts as a major coordinator of adaptive responses to cognitively perceived stressful stimuli[31]. There is also evidence for CRH hypersecretion in depression and, as noted above, this forms part of the basis for current concepts of limbic system-hypothalamic dysregulation being responsible for the increased HPA activity seen in affective disorder[5]. Some authors have gone further and suggested that hypersecretion of CRH alone may account for the characteristic symptoms of depression[32] (although, as Murphy[4] points out, this would not explain the presence of similar symptoms in the depression associated with Cushing's syndrome where CRH levels are reduced). In the rat, CRH induces many behavioural changes, including fear of new situations, increased locomotion, and decreased social interaction, food consumption, sexual receptivity and responding in conflict tests[33]. In healthy human controls, the administration of CRH produces many of the changes in the sleep EEG and sleep-associated hormone secretion that are seen in depression[31].

Evidence for CRH hypersecretion in depression is indirect: CSF levels of CRH are increased in depression[32] and postmortem studies show that CRH binding sites in the frontal cortex of suicide victims are reduced compared to controls, consistent with down-regulation of CRH binding sites in the presence of CRH hypersecretion[34]. Plasma levels of ACTH in depression have been found to be high in some studies[35] but low or normal in most others[36]. This has been suggested by some authors to indicate the outcome of opposing effects of CRH stimulation versus glucocorticoid feedback inhibition of the pituitary corticotroph[31]. Others suggest the possibility of pituitary stimulants of corticosteroid secretion other than ACTH in depression[4], although it has been shown that CRH has a direct action on the adrenal, potentiating the effect of low levels of ACTH[37]. There is agreement that administration of CRH to depressed patients results in a reduced ACTH response but a normal cortisol response compared to controls[5,38]. This abnormal response to CRH in depressed patients is seen even in the absence of raised cortisol levels[39], suggesting that a defect of negative feedback alone does not account for the altered HPA activity in depression.

Recently the validity of the dexamethasone suppression test in depression has been questioned on the grounds of both altered dexamethasone pharmacokinetics in depression[40] and its lack of suitability for evaluating the contribution of the limbic system to HPA abnormalities in depression[41]. This latter point is an important one: dexamethasone does not bind to hippocampal corticosteroid receptors in vivo[42], and may therefore in exerting its principal feedback effects at the pituitary rather than brain be behaving quite differently from endogenous corticosteroids. This has led to the development of several new dynamic tests which are proposed as probes of suprapituitary components of HPA axis regulation in depression. Young and coworkers demonstrated that intravenous infusion of cortisol resulted in fast-feedback inhibition of corticotroph secretion of β endorphin/β lipotropin in normal controls but had no effect in depressed patients[41]. Because fast feedback inhibition is thought to involve hippocampal corticosteroid receptors in the rat (see above) they interpret this finding as supporting the concept of abnormal hippocampal regulation of CRH in depression. This group have also suggested the use of corticosterone instead of dexamethasone as a suppression test, as corticosterone, a minor endogenous corticosteroid in the human, is known to bind to hippocampal receptors, unlike dexamethasone[43]. It remains to be seen whether this elegant idea has a practical application in the elucidation of suprapituitary and limbic elements in corticosteroid feedback in depression.

The best documented of the recently introduced tests of suprapituitary elements of the HPA axis is the combined dexamethasone-hCRH test, developed by Holsboer and coworkers[31]. In normal controls dexamethasone reduces the amount of ACTH released in response to CRH, due to negative feedback at the pituitary level. In depressed patients, however, dexamethasone premedication enhances the ACTH response to CRH, rather than suppressing it[31,44]. The authors postulate that this reflects impaired inhibition by brain corticosteroid receptors of hypothalamic ACTH secretagogues, and ascribe this impaired inhibition to down regulation of brain corticosteroid receptors in response to hypercortisolaemia in depression. Regardless of its mechanism of action, the combined dexamethasone-hCRH test has been shown to be a sensitive indicator of HPA abnormalities in depression. Although the response to this test gradually normalizes with euthymia, the process of normalization becomes prolonged and frequently incomplete with increasing age[31]. Furthermore, the amount of cortisol secreted in response to the dexamethasone-hCRH test increases with age in patients who experience repeated episodes of major depression, but not in controls[45]. This may reflect a progressive inability to terminate the stress response appropriately as predicted by the glucocorticoid cascade hypothesis[2].

Effects of the treatment of depression on the HPA axis

With successful treatment of depression there is normalization of plasma cortisol, response to the dexamethasone suppression test and response to the CRH test[4]. There have been several studies showing that antidepressant drugs have effects on brain corticosteroid receptors. Pepin and coworkers[46] described small increases in GR in rat primary neuron culture in response to tricyclic antidepressants. More recently, a variety of drugs including imipramine, desipramine, ketanserin and lithium have all been shown to increase GR mRNA in different regions of rat brain[47]. There are some surprising sex differences in this study, which the authors ascribe to sex differences in central neurotransmitter systems. It is of note that imipramine increased GR in both the hypothalamus and hippocampus of male and female rats, but that desipramine in the female rat and lithium in the male rat had no effect on GR mRNA. A less confusing report by Seckl and Fink[48] describes large increases in both GR and MR mRNA in the hippocampus but not the cortex of male rats treated for 14 days with either amitriptyline or desipramine. In conjunction with their previous report that lesions of central serotonergic systems decrease the expression of GR and MR mRNA in subregions of the hippocampus[26], Seckl and Fink suggest that antidepressants, acting via increased monoamine levels to increase hippocampal corticosteroid receptor number, may restore the sensitivity of the HPA to corticosteroid feedback, resulting in normalization of HPA activity. This effect may not be dependent on monoamine mediation, as Pepin et al.[46] also showed that tricyclic antidepressants were able to activate the GR gene promoter directly. It is of interest to note that repeated electrically induced seizures in the rat caused a similar selective increase in hippocampal GR receptors, despite also increasing corticosteroid levels[49]. These findings merit further study, as a specific action of antidepressants and ECT in normalizing the HPA axis would have profound implications for our understanding of the role of HPA dysfunction in the pathophysiology of depression.

Future areas of research in the HPA axis in depression

While there remains huge scope for future research aimed at increasing our understanding of the limbic-hypothalamic-pituitary adrenal system in depression and in the implications of this for antidepressant treatment, there are two other areas of interest which are worthy of mention. These are the interaction between neuroendocrine and immune systems in depression, and the possible contribution of corticosteroids other than cortisol in the pathophysiology of affective disorders. These areas remain speculative, but of considerable potential importance.

Neuroendocrine–immune interactions in depression The interaction between the CNS and the immune system is well documented, and some authors have extended this to the concept of a bidirectional regulatory interaction between the immune system and the HPA[50,51]. Glucocorticoids have many, mostly suppressive, effects on the immune system as part of their role in preventing damaging overactivity of the stress response[52]. In turn, several cytokines produced by stimulated immune cells are able to stimulate the HPA axis[51]. The best studied of these interactions is the HPA stimulation induced by interleukin 1_β (IL 1β) which is released from activated macrophages and acts principally at the hypothalamus to stimulate CRH[53]. A closed regulatory loop is formed by the resulting increased levels of glucocorticoid acting to inhibit macrophage secretion of IL 1β and to alter the differentiation and function of the monocyte-macrophage cell line[54].

These complex interactions between the immune system and the HPA axis are of considerable interest in depression where there is HPA overactivity: first, they allow the use of immunocytes as peripheral models of the central actions of glucocorticoid excess (as described above); and secondly, they predict that immunological competency may be impaired in depression, providing a potential link between depression and increased risk of immune-related diseases such as infections, autoimmune disorders and cancer. Early studies of immune function in depression have produced conflicting results, partly ascribed to methodological problems[55]. Currently, there are indications that natural killer cell activity is altered[56] and that some elements of impaired immune function in depression correlate with HPA axis activity[57]. However, it remains the case that no clear link has been established between depression, impaired immunity and increased physical ill health, leading Stein et al.[55] to describe the reported immune changes in depression as 'findings in search of meaning'. Overall, further research is needed to produce empirical evidence to support an attractive theoretical concept.

The role of corticosteroids other than cortisol in depression Despite the large number of circulating corticosteroids and their metabolites, some of which are known to be increased in depression and many of which are known to have effects on brain function and behaviour[4], attention in depression has focused almost entirely on cortisol. Recently, however, considerable interest has been provoked by the demonstration that several classes of corticosteroids can exert immediate effects at the membrane level[58] rather than through conventional cytosolic receptors with a delayed effect at the level of the genome. Pregnane steroids such as 3α-hydroxy-dihydroprogesterone (3α-OH-DHP) and 3α-tetrahydro-deoxycorticosterone have long been known to act as potent endogenous anaesthetic and narcotic agents[59] and have now been shown to potentiate the actions of GABA at the $GABA_A$ receptor[58]. Early studies used relatively high concentrations of corticosteroids, implying a pharmacological effect, but similar effects have been reported using picomolar concentrations of 3α-OH-DHP[60], suggesting that this corticosteroid, at least, may be a physiologically relevant modulator of GABAergic neurotransmission. Two other corticosteroids, dehydroepiandrosterone (DHEA) and pregnenolone, have been shown to inhibit GABAergic transmission in their sulphated forms, and have been termed 'neurosteroids' as there is evidence that they may be synthesized by brain tissue as well as by the adrenal cortex[61]. The significance of these recent findings is not yet known. Surprisingly, the role of these corticosteroids in depression has never been studied, despite evidence that they may affect behaviour and mood[4].

A recent series of reports[62] has added a newly discovered corticosteroid to the list of those which may have a role in affective disorder: ouabain. In these studies, Hamlyn and colleagues report the isolation and characterization of an endogenous ouabain-like factor which is indistinguishable from the plant steroid ouabain, and which appears to be a product of the human adrenal cortex[63]. Like ouabain, this endogenous ouabain-like compound was a potent inhibitor of Na^+/K^+-ATPase. Abnormal membrane transport is one of the most reliable of the biological markers for bipolar affective disorder[64], and many studies have described impaired Na^+/K^+-ATPase activity in both manic and depressed patients[65,66]. In addition, a high Na^+/K^+-ATPase activity in patients with bipolar affective disorder is associated with good prognosis over the following year, and lithium restores Na^+/K^+-ATPase activity to control levels[67]. Different elements of Na^+/K^+-ATPase activity show both state- and trait-dependent abnormalities[68]. However, not all studies are in agreement, with reports of both no difference in Na^+/K^+-ATPase activity between patients and controls and increased Na^+/K^+-ATPase activity in mania and depression[64]. Hokin-Neaverson and Jefferson[67] suggest that some of these discrepancies may have been caused by the existence of an endogenous inhibitor of Na^+/K^+-ATPase whose effect on measurable activity would depend on the methodology used, and whose levels in plasma may be variable. The adrenal endogenous ouabain-like compound described above would be an obvious candidate for mediating some of the effects on Na^+/K^+-ATPase seen in bipolar affective disorder, given both its effects as an inhibitor of Na^+/K^+-ATPase and the generally increased output of adrenocortical steroids in affective disorders.

Further studies are needed on the control of secretion of endogenous ouabain-like compound, and the way in which this is altered in affective disorder. The potential importance of this compound lies in the close similarities between mechanisms of Na^+/K^+ transport in erythrocytes and excitable membranes and in the role of Na^+/K^+-ATPase in amino acid precursor uptake and neurotransmitter reuptake in nervous tissue. It is of note that the Na^+/K^+-ATPase isomer present in brain appears to have a higher affinity for ouabain than that present in the erythrocyte[69]. Finally, it is tempting to speculate on the role of the interaction of a humoral agent determined by the neuroendocrine environment with a potentially genetically determined trait abnormality of Na^+/K^+-ATPase[66] in the pathogenesis of bipolar affective disorder.

Applications of neuroendocrine probes in affective disorders

Neuroendocrine challenge tests form part of the armamentarium for the assessment of central neural function in patients in a clinical setting. A neuroendocrine 'probe' involves the administration of a drug which penetrates into the brain and activates central neurones, thereby regulating the release of hypothalamo-pituitary hormones which can be detected in the peripheral circulation. The size of the hormonal response provides an estimate of the sensitivity of the probe-responsive neural inputs to the hypothalamus, and reflects the integration of pre- and postsynaptic influences on overall functional neurotransmission.

We will discuss the 5HT probes which have been applied in depressed patients, and the recent advances in the development of novel challenge tests with greater pharmacological specificity for 5HT systems.

5HT and depression

Evidence for brain 5HT dysfunction in depressed patients has accumulated through several lines of study. CSF 5-hydroxy-indoleacetic acid (5HIAA) concentrations are reduced, platelet imipramine binding sites are reduced and $5HT_2$ binding sites in brain are increased in most, but not all[70], post-mortem studies. Plasma tryptophan and brain tryptophan availability (as reflected by the tryptophan to neutral amino acid ratio) are also reduced. Drugs which increase intrasynaptic 5HT by inhibiting presynaptic 5HT uptake alleviate depression. However, the functional and therapeutic significance of all these serotonergic changes remains controversial. Serotonergic neuroendocrine probes can be applied both to explore the functional status of 5HT systems in depressed patients and also to assess the effect of antidepressant treatments on 5HT neurotransmission in a clinical setting.

Serotonergic agents and neuroendocrine secretion in normal man

All the neuroendocrine probes which have been applied in human studies enhance serotonergic neurotransmission by a variety of mechanisms. 5-hydroxytryptophan (5-HTP) and L-tryptophan (LTP) are precursors of 5HT. Clomipramine is an inhibitor of presynaptic 5HT re-uptake. m-Chlorophenylpiperazine (mCPP), MK-212 and the azopirones (gepirone, buspirone and ipsaperone) are direct 5HT receptor agonists.

LTP and 5HTP Oral LTP and 5HTP have inconsistent effects on secretion of anterior pituitary hormones in normal volunteers. Reasons for this include the marked variability in absorption between subjects and the frequency of stressful side effects, especially nausea, which is likely to be a nonspecific stimulus for hormone secretion. For these reasons, the oral route has fallen into disuse. However, intravenous LTP and 5HTP reliably stimulate prolactin and growth hormone secretion[71,72] and LTP in particular has been adopted extensively as a neuroendocrine challenge in patient studies. One drawback is their lack of specificity. They also activate catecholaminergic neurones and it has not been possible to demonstrate consistent inhibition of endocrine responses with 5HT antagonists such as cyproheptadine and ketanserin.

Fenfluramine Oral DL-fenfluramine consistently stimulates prolactin and ACTH/cortisol secretion in man, while effects on growth hormone are inconsistent[73]. However, DL-fenfluramine, like the 5HT precursors, lacks 5HT specificity and also has presynaptic releasing activity at dopaminergic and noradrenergic neurones. In addition, it causes unpleasant side effects including dysphoria, abdominal pain and anxiety, which are potent nonspecific stimuli for endocrine secretion.

The recent availability of the stereo-isomer D-fenfluramine has been an important development. It is more specific for serotonergic pathways[74] and is much better tolerated, causing mild sedation and anorexia, and occasional headaches, which are less likely to confound specific probe-induced neuroendocrine effects. D-fenfluramine thus offers distinct pharmacological advantages and holds great promise for application in patient studies.

Clomipramine and fluvoxamine Intravenous clomipramine (25 mg) reliably stimulates prolactin secretion. Growth hormone responses are more variable with only about 50% of subjects exhibiting a response, and this is likely to be related to nausea. Side effects can be reduced without loss of the prolactin stimulant effect by the use of a lower dose (10 mg)[75]. However, a further limitation to the utility of clomipramine as a probe is that its major metabolite desmethyldesipramine has noradrenergic activity. Theoretically the selective serotonin reuptake inhibitors (SSRI) such as fluvoxamine and fluoxetine have potential as probes with greater serotonergic specificity. Although a prolactin response can be demonstrated in animal studies, oral fluvoxamine does not stimulate prolactin secretion in man and intravenous preparations of the SSRIs are not available for use in patients at present.

Direct 5HT agonists The 5HT precursors and the 5HT releasing and reuptake inhibiting agents stimulate 5HT neurotransmission by enhancing presynaptic 5HT availability, and thus depend on intact presynaptic mechanisms to exert their postsynaptic effect. The direct agonists are not constrained by this proviso and can potentially be used to discriminate between pre- and post-synaptic receptor-mediated function.

Buspirone, ipsaperone and gepirone are promising new azapirone probes for the assessment of $5HT_{1a}$ receptor-mediated function in man. Buspirone and gepirone cause a dose dependent rise in prolactin, growth hormone and cortisol secretion involving pre- and postsynaptic $5HT_{1a}$ activation[76,77].

However, buspirone also binds to D_2 dopamine receptors and neuroendocrine responses may be mediated by D_2 blockade. Gepirone has the advantage of being more specific for $5HTI_a$ receptors[77], although it may also have partial DA agonist activity. The nausea associated with gepirone correlates with cortisol secretion, raising the possibility that nonspecific stress is a confounding influence. Despite these reservations, these agents hold considerable promise in terms of assessing 5HT function in humans.

Oral administration of MK-212 produces a dose-dependent increase in cortisol and prolactin which may depend on activation of $5HT_{1c}$ and $5HT_2$ receptor mechanisms. This compound merits study in patients because of its 5HT specificity, although side effects may limit its full potential as a specific probe[78].

M-chlorophenylpiperazine (MCPP) is a metabolite of trazodone which stimulates prolactin and cortisol secretion in normal man, a process which is likely to involve activation of $5HT_{1a}$, $5HT_{1c}$ and $5HT_2$ receptor mechanisms[79]. It is not specific to serotonergic receptors, having potent affinity for alpha$_2$ adrenoceptors as well. Another limitation is the frequency of stressful side effects including nausea, anxiety and sometimes panic.

From the above considerations of the currently available neuroendocrine probes of 5HT neurotransmission, it can be seen that, whilst there are several newly available 5HT specific probes, there is also scope for development and introduction of alternative probes.

Neuroendocrine probe studies in depressed patients

5HT precursors Westerberg et al.[80] administered oral 5HTP, with a carboxylase inhibitor to enhance its availability in brain, and failed to demonstrate any consistent hormone responses in either depressed patients or controls. In contrast, Meltzer et al.[81] elicited enhanced cortisol responses in both depressed and manic patients. This may be interpreted as reflecting a compensatory postsynaptic hypersensitivity secondary to a presynaptic 5HT deficiency and could be consistent with the increase of $5HT_2$ receptor demonstrated in postmortem studies of depression.

Prolactin responses to LTP are attenuated in depressed patients, suggesting that 5HT neurotransmission may be impaired[82]. However, more recent studies have emphasized the important influence of weight loss on these neuroendocrine responses. Weight loss is associated with enhanced prolactin responses and attenuated responses were only seen in depressed patients who had lost less than 3 kg in weight[83]. The size of the prolactin response was also highly inversely correlated with basal cortisol concentrations. Hypercortisolaemia may attenuate the prolactin response to LTP by reducing $5HT_1$ receptor function[83]. Price et al.[84] found that enhanced prolactin responses in melancholic and psychotically depressed patients could be accounted for by high basal prolactin concentrations, although the influence of cortisol levels was not determined. In this large study involving 126 patients, few had experienced significant weight loss. Thus weight loss, hypercortisolemia and hyperprolactinemia need to be taken into account when interpreting studies of the LTP-prolactin response in depression.

5HT releasers and reuptake inhibitors Several groups have demonstrated attenuated prolactin responses to DL-fenfluramine in depressed patients[85]. However, Asnis et al.[86] found normal responses whilst Mitchell and Smythe[87] described an attenuated prolactin response which was restricted to the endogenous subtype and was partially dependent on basal prolactin and cortisol concentrations. This again emphasizes the importance of accounting for basal hormone concentrations in interpreting neurohormonal responses. Depressed patients have impaired prolactin responses to clomipramine[88] and the more specific serotonergic agent D-fenfluramine[89].

5HT receptor agonists Neuroendocrine responses to MCPP in depressed patients are normal[90]. However, ipsaperone-induced ACTH/cortisol responses are attenuated suggesting impairment of $5HT_{1a}$ receptor-mediated function[91].

Further studies using specific receptor subtype probes are needed, but, on balance, the neuroendocrine evidence favours an impairment in 5HT neurotransmission in depressed patients.

Antidepressant treatments and 5HT neuroendocrine probes
Concurrent antidepressant medication has significant effects on neuroendocrine responsivity and the medication status of patients needs to be carefully considered. In practice, it is very difficult to study unmedicated depressed patients since they are very likely to be taking chronic prophylactic treatment or have started treatment prior to referral to hospital. Conventionally drug-free intervals prior to neuroendocrine testing are between 1 and 3 weeks. However, drug effects may last much longer. For example, the growth hormone response to clonidine may be blunted for several months following antidepressant withdrawal[92] and the prolactin response to L-tryptophan is enhanced 2 weeks after discontinuation of amitriptyline[93]. Further studies are needed to determine how long drug effects may persist after stopping treatment, in order to distinguish primary changes in 5HT sensitivity from treatment effects in patients.

The sensitivity of neuroendocrine tests to antidepressant medication can, however, be usefully applied to explore the important unanswered question of how antidepressant efficacy relates to serotonergic neurotransmission. Chronic treatment with SSRIs causes a) down-regulation of postsynaptic $5HT_2$ receptors which would reduce 5HT neurotransmission, b) down regulation of $5HT_{1a}$ autoreceptors which would increase 5HT neurotransmission and c) up regulation of postsynaptic $5HT_1$ receptors which would increase 5HT neuronal activity[94]. Electrophysiological studies suggest that chronic antidepressant treatment enhances 5HT neurotransmission, whilst some 5HT-mediated behaviours are attenuated. Sequential neuroendocrine challenges provide one way of assessing the overall functional effect of antidepressant treatment on 5HT neurotransmission in man. Shapira et al.[95] have shown that the prolactin responses to fenfluramine are enhanced after 3 weeks treatment with imipramine, whilst the prolactin response to tryptophan is also sensitized by chronic antidepressant treatment both in patients[93] and in normal controls[96].

Fluvoxamine treatment enhances the prolactin response to LTP more rapidly than does desipramine, which is consistent with its greater 5HT potency. In patients with obsessive compulsive disorder, ACTH/cortisol and hypothermic responses to ipsaperone were attenuated after 3 months treatment with fluvoxamine, suggesting that therapeutic effects may be mediated through desensitization of $5HT_{1a}$ receptor-mediated systems[97]. Similar studies in depressed patients are awaited with interest.

In animals, 5HT release is increased by acute, and reduced by chronic, lithium treatment. 5HT autoreceptors are also desensitized by chronic treatment. Thus, whilst short-term treatment enhances 5HT neurotransmission, the adaptational effects of chronic treatment restores 5HT neurotransmission to pretreatment levels. Neuroendocrine studies in patients reflect these findings. Short-term lithium enhances 5HT mediated neuroendocrine responses to fenfluramine, tryptophan and clomipramine, while longer-term treatment normalizes neuroendocrine responses[98]. However, lithium augmentation of tricyclic antidepressant treatment in patients with resistant depression enhanced prolactin responses to tryptophan over a 4 week period, although this increased 5HT mediated activity did not clearly correlate with clinical response[99].

Enhancement of 5HT function is not confined to pharmacological antidepressant treatments since ECT has similar effects, causing enhanced prolactin responses to DL-fenfluramine[100]. Systematic studies of the newly available specific 5HT probes in depressed patients, both before and after antidepressant treatments, will allow further exploration of the relationship between 5HT neurotransmission and antidepressant efficacy.

State- and trait-dependent neuroendocrine change

A neuroendocrine abnormality may be state dependent (that is confined to periods of active illness and normalizing in parallel with improvement in symptoms) or trait dependent (enduring through periods of remission). The distinction between state and trait markers is particularly relevant in discriminating between changes of potential etiological significance and nonspecific influences of epiphenomena such as weight loss. Trait abnormalities are likely to reflect enduring dysfunction which may promote vulnerability to relapse.

The search for neuroendocrine trait markers requires tenacity because of the difficulty in finding patients who are both free of symptoms and psychotropic medication. However, the growth hormone response to clonidine was attenuated in patients who had fully recovered from an episode of endogenous depression and been medication free for between 4 weeks and 4 years, suggesting that alpha$_2$ adrenoceptor mediated function may be persistently reduced[101]

Although Numberger et al.[102] found blunted tryptophan induced ACTH and cortisol responses in euthymic bipolar patients, some had only been withdrawn from medication for 2 weeks, making it difficult to determine whether this is a trait abnormality independent of residual effects of medication. In a study of 5HT function using the prolactin and GH responses to LTP, Upadahyaya et al.[103] tested patients at least 3 months after recovery and cessation of antidepressant treatment, by which time neuroendocrine responses had normalized, after taking into account effects of weight loss.

Future studies

Neuroendocrine challenge tests constitute a valuable method of assessing functional neurotransmission in patients. The importance of matching variables such as age, sex and menstrual cycle stage[104] between patient and normal control groups is now fully recognized. We are also aware of the need to correct for confounding influences such as weight loss, stress and medication status when interpreting neuroendocrine probe studies.

We need probes with high 5HT selectivity which induce significant dose-dependent endocrine responses without stressful side effects. Further receptor-specific agonists and antagonists are needed which can be given to humans (for example, 5HT$_{1a}$ antagonists) in order to define the receptor subtype mechanisms involved in 5HT probes. We will then be able to use 5HT probes to explore more precisely the status of 5HT receptor subtypes in depression and how psychotropic treatments influence this.

Neurohormonal aspects of puerperal psychosis

Neuroendocrine challenge tests have recently been fruitfully developed and applied to explore the etiological basis of puerperal psychosis. Childbirth is a potent trigger of psychotic illness, with admission rates rising 20-fold during the first month after delivery. Puerperal psychosis is rare in the general population, complicating approximately 0.05–0.1% of deliveries. However, women who have a history of nonpuerperal or puerperal bipolar manic depressive psychosis are very vulnerable, with a 50% chance of relapsing in the first 6 weeks postpartum. The period of maximum risk is very soon after delivery, between the 4th and 14th postpartum day. Thus in vulnerable groups there is a predictable high risk of relapse within a narrow time frame in relation to the event of childbirth, and the event and relapse are separated by a symptom-free period of a few days. Puerperal psychosis therefore provides a model for the prospective study of biological mechanisms operating immediately before the onset of symptoms and before the need for psychotropic medication which would confound data interpretation. Biological triggers are likely to be of primary relevance in puerperal relapse of bipolar manic depressive psychosis since, in contrast to postpartum unipolar depression, there is no strong relationship between relapse and adverse life events[105].

Childbirth triggers a maternal endocrinological revolution. The fetoplacental unit synthesizes a variety of peptide growth factors and glycoprotein hormones, principally placental lactogen and human chorionic gonadotrophin. The sudden fall in concentrations of these factors is unlikely to be relevant as they do not cross the blood brain barrier. The fetoplacental unit has also commandeered the role of the maternal ovary such that its expulsion causes a 200-fold decrease in maternal plasma concentration of estrogen and progesterone over 2 days. Estrogen is particularly likely to be relevant to manic depressive relapse since it readily enters the brain where it binds to specific binding sites concentrated in limbic forebrain areas, particularly the hypothalamus, amygdala and hippocampus[106].

Immunocytochemical studies have recently permitted the visualization of estrogen receptors (ER) through pregnancy and the puerperium in the mouse. This technique has a great advantage over earlier autoradiographic studies because it obviates the need for gonadectomy to reduce competitive binding by endogenous estrogens. The density of estrogen binding sites is reduced in the hippocampus and hypothalamus in the puerperium relative to pregnancy[107]. The ER is intranuclear and, after estrogen binding, the complex interacts with sites on DNA to regulate mRNA expression and peptide synthesis. This process takes place over a time course which parallels the period between childbirth and psychotic relapse.

A neuroendocrine model of central estrogen receptor mediated function has been developed to explore whether the changes in ER associated with the puerperium in animals are paralleled in women and, if so, how these effects relate to psychotic relapse. In response to estrogen administration, estrogen sensitive neurophysin (ESN) is synthesized as part of a precursor preprooxytocin in cells in the anterior hypothalamus which contain ER[108]. The precursor is cleaved during transportation down the neurohypophyseal stalk and secreted from the neurohypophysis in equimolar amounts with oxytocin. It has no clear biological function following secretion and seems likely to act as a stabilizing carrier protein for oxytocin prior to its secretion into the peripheral circulation. ESN is more stable than oxytocin in plasma and can thus be more conveniently estimated. In normal women, there is a dose dependent ESN response to oral ethinylestradiol administration[109]. Following a single dose of 50 μg, ESN secretion is enhanced over a period of 5 days, which is consistent with an estrogen-induced genomic activation of protein synthesis. In normal puerperal women this response is attenuated during the first 2 postpartum weeks and by 1 month is normalizing[109]. Women with chronic estrogen deficiency in association with anorexia nervosa[109] and the menopause[110] have normal ESN responses to ethinylestradiol. This suggests that the attenuated postpartum ESN response is not simply a reflection of low ambient estrogen concentrations, but is more likely to reflect a specific effect of the rapid fluctuation in estrogen concentration on ER-mediated neuro-endocrine events. Studies are in progress to determine whether a change in ER mediated function as reflected by the ESN response in the early postpartum period is predictive of bipolar relapse in high risk women, and whether estrogen treatment immediately after delivery will prevent relapse.

The link between puerperal associated changes in estrogen mediated events and psychotic relapse is likely to involve neurotransmitter systems[111], and dopamine is one likely candidate. Estrogen treatment down-regulates striatal D2 receptors[112] whilst estrogen withdrawal enhances dopamine mediated behaviours[113]. Wieck et al.[114] have applied a neuroendocrine probe of dopamine receptor mediated function (the growth hormone response to apomorphine, which reflects D2 dopamine receptor activation) in women at high risk of puerperal relapse by virtue of their past history of bipolar manic depressive psychosis. Women were tested 4 days postpartum when they were still largely symptom free and taking no medication. Of the 15 women tested, the 8 who relapsed had enhanced growth hormone responses compared with both the control group and those who were vulnerable but remained well. Thus dopaminergic hyperactivity, perhaps induced by estrogen withdrawal, may trigger relapse in women at risk, suggesting that estrogen treatment may prevent relapse by reducing DA receptor mediated sensitivity.

Women who have had puerperal psychosis may suffer nonpuerperal relapses just prior to their menstrual period, a time when estrogen concentrations are falling[115]. In normal women, dopamine receptor mediated function fluctuates throughout the menstrual cycle[116]. In high risk women it may be even more sensitive to cyclical estrogen fluctuations during the menstrual cycle as well as postpartum. Studies are in progress to test this hypothesis.

Neuroendocrine studies in puerperal psychosis have provided valuable information on the functional status of central neurotransmitter systems and a rationale for ongoing studies of prophylactic hormone treatment in patients.

Endocrine aspects of neurodevelopment and cognitive function

We have described recent developments in our understanding of neuro-endocrine processes in psychiatric disorders, using as examples the pathophysiological role of the HPA in depression, and the use of neuro-endocrine probes both in the assessment of 5HT function in health and in depression and in investigating the hormonal basis of puerperal psychosis. All of this body of knowledge is based on what may be termed 'activational' effects of hormones on the mature adult brain. There is also, however, growing interest in both the 'organizational' effects of hormones on the developing brain[117] and the effects of early environment on adult neuroendocrine function[118]. These are exciting areas of neuroendocrine research with implications for our understanding of the role hormones may play in the etiology of psychiatric disorder.

Animal studies have shown that gonadal steroids, in particular, have a critical role in the organization of neuronal systems responsible for neuro-endocrine functions[119], and influence the development of both cerebral laterality[120] and sexual dimorphism[121] in the brain. In the human, cognitive processes in the adult are sensitive to both varying levels of endogenous gonadal steroids[122] and administration of exogenous steroids[123]. There is also growing evidence that the endocrine environment to which the developing human brain is subjected can influence the development of the observed sex differences in human behavioural and cognitive processes[121]. Thus gonadal steroids have been implicated in the development of sex differences in behavioural and cognitive processes at two critical periods: permanent organizational effects on brain differentiation during gestation and shortly after birth; and temporary activational effects on these differentiated areas from puberty onwards[124]. We can postulate that the biological contribution to the gender effect in susceptibility to psychiatric disorder may be partly due to neurodevelopmental factors in addition to the effects of prevailing gonadal steroid levels.

Animal studies have also provided evidence of the way in which early environment can affect the development of neuroendocrine systems and so determine the adult neuroendocrine response to environmental stressors. Rats that are handled during the first 3 weeks of life show decreased fearful-ness of new environments and a reduced HPA response to a variety of stressors throughout life[118]. Recently, it has been demonstrated that neonatal handling causes a permanent and specific increase in hippocampal GR, resulting in increased sensitivity of the HPA to negative feedback by circulat-ing corticosteroids[118]. The ability to terminate the glucocorticoid stress

J A Bearn and P W Raven

response rapidly in these rats represents an adaptation to a stressful environment and appears to afford some protection against the cognitive decline due to hippocampal damage seen in aged rats subject to chronic stress[125]. It can also be envisaged that the reduced magnitude of their glucocorticoid response to stress may render these rats more susceptible to other pathological processes.

In conclusion, we have described several ways in which circulating levels of steroid hormones respond to environmental changes and how their effects are exerted by allowing expression of parts of the genome. This represents a model for the interaction between genes and environment which will facilitate the study of neuroendocrine factors which protect against and predispose to psychiatric disorder.

References

(1) McEwen BS, Angulo J, Cameron H et al. Paradoxical effects of adrenal steroids on the brain: Protection versus degeneration. *Biol Psychiat* 1992; 31: 177–99.

(2) Sapolsky RM, Krey LC, McEwen BS. The neuroendocrinology of stress and aging: the glucocorticoid cascade hypothesis. *Endocr Rev.* 1986; 7: 284–301.

(3) Nemeroff CB, Krishnan RR, Reed D et al. Adrenal gland enlargement in major depression. *Arch Gen Psychiat* 1992; 49: 384–7.

(4) Murphy BEP. Steroids and depression. *J Steroid Biochem Molec Biol* 1991; 38: 537–59.

(5) Amsterdam JD, Maislin G, Gold P, Winokur A. The assessment of abnormalities in hormonal responsiveness at multiple levels of the hypothalamic-pituitary-adrenocortical axis in depressive illness. *Psychoneuroendocrinology* 1989; 14: 43–62.

(6) Reul JMHM, de Kloet ER. Two receptor systems for corticosterone in rat brain: microdistribution and differential occupation. *Endocrinology* 1985; 117: 2505–11.

(7) Miesfeld R, Okret S, Wikstrom A-C et al. Characterization of a steroid hormone receptor gene and mRNA in wild-type and mutant cells. *Nature* 1984; 312: 779–81.

(8) Hollenberg SM, Weinberger C, Ong ES et al. Primary structure and expression of a functional human glucocorticoid receptor cDNA. *Nature* 1983; 318: 635–41.

(9) Arriza JL, Weinberger C, Cerelli G et al. Cloning of human mineralocorticoid receptor complementary DNA: structural and functional kinship with the glucocorticoid receptor. *Science* 1987; 237:268–75.

(10) Patel PD, Sherman TG, Goldman DJ, Watson SJ. Molecular cloning of a mineralocorticoid (type I) receptor complementary DNA from rat hippocampus. *Mol Endocrinol* 1990; 3: 1877–85.

(11) Chao HM, Choo PH, McEwen BS. Glucocorticoid and mineralocorticoid receptor mRNA expression in rat brain. *Neuroendocrinology* 1989; 50: 365–71.

(12) Seckl JR, Dickson KL, Yates C, Fink G. Distribution of glucocorticoid and

mineralocorticoid receptor messenger RNA expression in human postmortem hippocampus. *Brain Res* 1991; 561: 332–7.

(13) Spencer RL, Young EA, Choo PH, McEwen BS. Adrenal steroid type I and type II receptor binding: estimates of in vivo receptor number, occupancy, and activation with varying level of steroid. *Brain Res* 1990; 514: 37–48.

(14) Jacobson L, Sapolsky R. The role of the hippocampus in feedback regulation of the hypothalamic-pituitary-adrenocortical axis. *Endocr Rev* 1991; 12: 118–34.

(15) Herman J, Schafer M, Young E, et al. Evidence for hippocampaı regulation of neuroendocrine neurons of hypothalamo-pituitary adrenocortical axis.*J. Neurosci* 189; 9: 3072–82.

(16) Magarinos A, Somoza G, DeNicola A. Glucocorticoid negative feedback and glucocorticoid receptors after hippocampectomy in rats. *Horm Metab Res* 1987; 19: 105–9.

(17) Pfeiffer A, Lapointe B, Barden N. Hormonal regulation of type II glucocorticoid receptor messenger ribonucleic acid in rat brain. *Endocrinology* 1991; 129: 2166–74.

(18) De Kloet ER, Sybesma H, Reul JMHM. Selective control by corticosterone of serotonin receptor capacity in the raphe-hippocampal system. *Neuroendocrinology* 1986; 42: 513–21.

(19) Mendelson SD, McEwen BS. Autoradiographic analyses of the effects of adrenalectomy and corticosterone on 5-HT$_{1A}$ and 5-HT$_{1B}$ receptors in the dorsal hippocampus and cortex of the rat. *Neuroendocrinology* 1992; 55: 444–50.

(20) Joels M, de Kloet ER. Coordinative mineralocorticoid and glucocorticoid receptor-mediated control of responses to serotonin in rat hippocampus. *Neuroendocrinology* 1992; 55: 344–50.

(21) Miller AL, Chaptal C, McEwen BS, Peck EJ. Modulation of high affinity GABA uptake into hippocampal synaptosomes by glucocorticoids. *Psychoneuroendocrinology* 1978; 3: 155–64.

(22) Roberts DC, Bloom FE. Adrenal steroid-induced changes in beta-adrenergic receptor binding in rat hippocampus. *Eur J Pharmac* 1981; 74: 37–41.

(23) Sapolsky RM. Glucocorticoids, hippocampal damage and the glutamatergic synapse. *Prog Brain Res* 1990; 86: 13–23.

(24) Veldhuis HD, de Kloet ER. Significance of ACTH$_{4-10}$ in the control of hippocampal corticosterone receptor capacity of hypophysectomized rats. *Neuroendocrinology* 1982; 34: 374–80.

(25) Meaney MJ, Aitken DH, Sapolsky RM. Thyroid hormones influence the development of hippocampal glucorticoid receptors in the rat: a mechanism for the effects of postnatal handling on the development of the adrenocortical stress response. *Neuroendocrinology* 1987; 45: 278–83.

(26) Seckl JR, Dickson KL, Fink G. Central 5,7-hydroxytryptamine lesions decrease hippocampal glucocorticoid and mineralocorticoid receptor messenger ribonucleic acid expression. *J Neuroendocrinol* 1990; 2; 911–6.

(27) Spencer RL, Miller AH, Stein M, McEwen BS. Corticosterone regulation of type I and type II adrenal steroid receptors in brain, pituitary, and immune tissue. *Brain Res* 1991; 549: 236–46.

(28) Lowy MT, Reder AT, Antel JP, Meltzer HY. Glucocorticoid resistance in

depression: the dexamethasone suppression test and lymphocyte sensitivity to dexamethasone. *Am J Psychiat* 1985; 141: 1365–7.

(29) Whalley LJ, Borthwick N, Copolov D, et al. Glucocorticoid receptors and depression. *Br Med J* 1986; 292: 859–61.

(30) Wassef A, Smith EM, Rose RM, et al. Mononuclear leukocyte glucocorticoid receptor binding characteristics and down-regulation in major depression. *Psychoneuroendocrinology* 1990; 15: 59–68.

(31) Holsboer F. The hypothalamic-pituitary-adrenocortical system. In Paykel ES, *Handbook of affective disorders*. Churchill Livingstone, 1992: 267–287.

(32) Roy A, Pickar D, Paul S et al. CSF corticotropin-releasing hormone in depressed patients and normal control subjects. *Am J Psychiat* 1987; 144: 641–5.

(33) Dunn AJ, Berridge CW. Physiological and behavioral responses to corticotropin-releasing factor administration: is CRF a mediator of anxiety or stress responses? *Brain Res Rev* 1990; 15: 71–100.

(34) Nemeroff CB, Owens MJ, Bissette G, et al. Reduced corticotropin-releasing factor binding sites in the frontal cortex of suicide victims. *Arch Gen Psychiat* 1988; 45: 577–9.

(35) Reus VI, Joseph M, and Dallman M. Regulation of ACTH and cortisol in depression. *Peptides* 1983; 4: 785–8.

(36) Linkowski P, Mendlewicz J, LeClerq R et al. The 24-hour profile of ACTH and cortisol in major depressive illness. *J Clin Endocr Metab* 1985; 61: 429–38.

(37) Tilders FJH, van Oers JWAM, Hinson JP. Corticotropin releasing factor controls corticosterone secretion from the rat adrenal gland. In Kvetnansky R, McCarty R & Axelrod J eds. *Stress: neurochemical and molecular advances*, eds. SA, New York, USA: Science Publishers, Gordon and Breach; 1992: 395–408.

(38) Holsboer F, von Bardeleben U, Gerken A et al. Blunted corticotropin and normal cortisol response to human corticotropin releasing factor (hCRF) in depression. *N Engl J Med* 1984; 311: 1127.

(39) Young EA, Watson SJ, Kotun J et al. β-lipotropin-β-endorphin response to low-dose ovine corticotropin releasing factor in endogenous depression. *Arch Gen Psychiat* 1990; 47:449–57.

(40) Maguire KP, Tuckwell VM, Schweitzer I et al. Dexamethasone kinetics in depressed patients before and after clinical response. *Psychoneuroendocrinology* 1990; 15: 113–23.

(41) Young EA, Haskett RF, Murphy-Weinberg V et al. Loss of glucocorticoid fast feedback in depression. *Arch Gen Psychiat* 1991; 48: 693–9.

(42) de Kloet ER, Wallach G, McEwen BS. Differences in corticosterone and dexamethasone binding to rat brain and pituitary. *Endocrinology* 1975; 76: 598–609.

(43) Haskett RF, Young EA, Murphy-Weinberg V. Use of corticosterone to assess glucocorticoid feedback mechanisms in depression. *Biol Psychiat* 1992; 31: 99A–100A.

(44) von Bardeleben U, Holsboer F. Cortisol response to a combined dexamethasone-human corticotropin-releasing hormone challenge in patients with depression. *J Neuroendocrinol* 1989; 1: 485–8.

(45) von Bardeleben U, Holsboer F. Effect of age on the cortisol response to human CRH in depressed patients pretreated with dexamethasone. *Biol Psychiat* 1991; 29: 1042–50.

(46) Pepin MC, Beaulieu S, Barden N. Antidepressants regulate glucocorticoids receptor messenger RNA concentrations in primary neuronal culture. *Mol Brain Res* 1989; 6: 77–83.

(47) Pfeiffer A, Veilleux S, Barden N. Antidepressant and other centrally acting drugs regulate glucocorticoid receptor messenger RNA levels in rat brain. *Psychoneuroendocrinology* 1991; 16: 505–15.

(48) Seckl JR, Fink G. Antidepressants increase glucocorticoid and mineralocorticoid receptor mRNA expression in rat hippocampus in vivo. *Neuroendocrinology* 1992; 55: 621–6.

(49) Young EA, Spencer RL, McEwen BS. Changes at multiple levels of the hypothalamo-pituitary adrenal axis following repeated electrically induced seizures. *Psychoneuroendocrinology* 1990; 15: 165–72.

(50) Bateman A, Singh A, Kral T, Solomon S. The immune-hypothalamic-pituitary-adrenal axis. *Endocr Rev* 1989; 10: 92–112.

(51) Buzzetti R, McLoughlin L, Scavo D, Rees LH. A critical assessment of the interactions between the immune system and the hypothalamo-pituitary-adrenal axis. *J Endrocrinol* 1989; 120: 183–7.

(52) Fauci AS. Immunosuppressive and anti-inflammatory effects of glucocorticoids. In Rousseau GG, Baxter JD, eds. *Glucocorticoid hormone action* New York: Springer; 1979: 449–465.

(53) Sapolsky R, Rivier C, Yamamoto G, et al. Interleukin-1 stimulates the secretion of hypothalamic corticotropin-releasing factor. *Science* 1987; 238: 522–4.

(54) Baybutt HN, Holsboer F. Inhibition of macrophage differentiation and function by cortisol. *Endocrinology* 1990; 127: 476–80.

(55) Stein M, Miller AH, Trestman RL. Depression, the immune system, and health and illness. *Arch Gen Psychiat* 1991; 48: 171–7.

(56) Evans DL, Folds JD, Petitto JM et al. Circulating natural killer cell phenotypes in men and women with major depression. *Arch Gen Psychiat* 1992; 49: 388–95.

(57) Maes M, Bosmans F, Suy F et al. A further exploration of the relationships between immune parameters and the HPA-axis activity in depressed patients. *Psychol Med* 1991; 21: 313–20.

(58) Majewska MD, Harrison NL, Schwartz RD et al. Steroid hormone metabolites are barbiturate-like modulators of the GABA receptor. *Science* 1986; 232: 1004–7.

(59) Selye H. Correlations between the chemical structure and the pharmacological actions of the steroids. *Endocrinology* 1942; 30: 437–53.

(60) Hiemke C, Jussofie A, Juptner M. Evidence that 3α-hydroxy-5α-pregnan-20-one is a physiologically relevant modulator of GABA-ergic neurotransmission. *Psychoneuroendocrinology* 1991; 16: 517–23.

(61) Baulieu E-E, Robel P. Neurosteroids: a new brain function? *J Steroid Biochem Molec Biol* 1990; 37: 395–403.

(62) Ludens JH, Clark MA, DuCharme DW et al. Purification of an endogenous digitalis-like factor from human plasma for structural analysis. *Hypertension* 1991; 17: 923–9.

(63) Editorial. Welcome to ouabain–a new steroid hormone. *Lancet* 1991; 338: 543–4.

(64) Meltzer HL. Is there a specific membrane defect in bipolar disorders? *Biol Psychiat* 1991; 30: 1071–4.

(65) Naylor GJ, Dick DAT, Dick EG et al. Erythrocyte membrane cation carrier in depressive illness. *Psychol Med* 1973; 3: 502–8.

(66) Hokin-Neaverson M, Jefferson JW. Erythrocyte sodium pump activity in bipolar affective disorder and other psychiatric disorders. *Neuropsychobiology* 1989; 22: 1–7.

(67) Hokin-Neaverson M, Jefferson J. Deficient erythrocyte NaK-ATPase activity in different affective states in bipolar affective disorder and normalization by lithium therapy. *Neuropsychobiology* 1989; 22: 18–25.

(68) Cowen PJ, Wood AJ. Biological markers of depression. *Psychol Med* 1991; 21: 831–6.

(69) Urayama O, Sweadner KJ. Ouabain sensitivity of alpha free isozyme of rat Na, K-ATPase. *Biochem Biophys Res Commun* 1988; 156: 796–800.

(70) Crow TJ, Cross AJ, Cooper SK et al. Neurotransmitter receptors and monoamine metabolites in the brains of patients with Alzheimer-type dementia and depression, and suicides. *Neuropharmacology* 1984; 23: 1561–9.

(71) Mashchak AC, Kletzky A, Spencer C, Artal LR. Transient effect of L-5-hydroxytryptophan on pituitary function in men and women. *Endocrinology* 1983; 56: 170–6.

(72) Charney DS, Heninger GR, Reinhard JF et al. The effect of IV L-tryptophan on prolactin, growth hormone and mood in healthy subjects. *Psychopharmacology* 1982; 77: 217–22.

(73) Mitchell PB, Smythe GA. Endocrine and amine responses to dl-fenfluramine in normal subjects. *Psychiat Res* 1991; 39: 141–53.

(74) Invernizzi R, Berettera C, Garattini S, Samanin R. D-and L-isomers of fenfluramine differ markedly in their interaction with brain serotonin and catecholamines in the rat. *Eur J Pharm* 1986; 120: 9–15.

(75) Golden RN, Hsiao JK, Lane E et al. The effects of intravenous clomipramine on neurohormones in healthy subjects. *J Clin Endocr Metab* 1989; 68: 632–7.

(76) Meltzer HY, Fleming R, Robertson A. The effect of buspirone on prolactin and growth hormone secretion in man. *Arch Gen Psychiat* 1983; 40: 1099–1102.

(77) Anderson IM, Cowen PJ, Graham-Smith DG. The effects of gepirone on neuroendocrine function and temperature in humans. *Psychopharmacology* 1990; 100: 498–503.

(78) Lowy MT, Meltzer HY. Stimulation of serum cortisol and prolactin secretion in humans by MK-212. *Biol Psychiat* 1988; 23: 818–28.

(79) Kahn RS and Wetzler S. m-Chlorophenylpiperazine as a probe of serotonin function. *Biol Psychiat* 1991; 30: 1139–1166.

(80) Westenberg HGM, Van Praag HM, De Jong TVM, Thijssen JHH. Postsynaptic serotonergic activity in depressive patients: evaluation of the neuroendocrine strategy. *Psychiat Res* 1982; 7: 361–71.

(81) Meltzer HY, Umberkoman-Witta B, Robertson A et al. Effect of 5-hydroxytryptophan on serum cortisol levels in major affective disorders. *Arch Gen Psychiat* 1984; 41: 366–74.

(82) Heninger GR, Charney DS, Sternberg DE. Serotonergic function in depres-

sion. Prolactin responses to intravenous tryptophan in depressed patients and healthy subjects. *Arch Gen Psychiat* 1984; 41: 398–402.

(83) Deakin JFW, Pennell I, Upadhyaya AJ, Lofthouse R. A neuroendocrine study of 5HT function in depression: evidence for biological mechanisms of endogenous and psychosocial causation. *Psychopharmacology* 1990; 101: 85–92.

(84) Price LH, Charney DS, Delgado PL, Heninger GR. Serotonin function and depression: neuroendocrine and mood responses to intravenous L-tryptophan in depressed patients and healthy comparison subjects. *Am J Psychiat* 1991; 148: 1518–25.

(85) Siever LJ, Murphy DL, Slater S et al. Plasma prolactin changes following fenfluramine in depressed patients compared to controls in depression. *Life Sci* 1984; 34: 1029–39.

(86) Asnis GM, Eisenberg J, Van Praag HM et al. The neuroendocrine response to fenfluramine in depressives and normal controls. *Biol Psychiat* 1988; 24: 117–20.

(87) Mitchell P, Smythe G. Hormonal responses to fenfluramine in depressed and control subjects. *J Affect Disorder* 1990; 19: 43–51.

(88) Golden RN, Hsiao JK, Lane E et al. Abnormal neuroendocrine responsivity to acute iv clomipramine challenge in depressed patients. *Psychiat Res* 1990; 31: 39–47.

(89) O'Keane V, Dinan TG. Prolactin and cortisol responses to d-fenfluramine in major depression: evidence for diminished responsivity of central serotonergic function. *Am J Psychiat* 1991; 148: 1009–15.

(90) Kahn RS, Wetzler S, Asnis GM et al. Serotonin receptor sensitivity in major depression. *Biol Psychiat* 1990; 28: 358–62.

(91) Lesch KP. $5HT_{1a}$ responsivity in anxiety disorders and depression. *Prog Neuro-psychopharmacol-Bio-Psychiat* 1991; 15: 723–33.

(92) Schittecatte M, Charles G, Machowske R. Tricyclic washout and growth hormone response to clonidine. *Br J. Psychiat* 1989; 154: 858–63.

(93) Charney DS, Heninger GR, Sternberg DE. Serotonin function and mechanism of action of antidepressant treatment: effects of amitriptyline and desipramine. *Arch Gen Psychiat* 1984; 41: 359–65.

(94) Marsden CA. The neuropharmacology of serotonin in the central nervous system. In: Feighner JP, Boyer WF, eds. *Selective serotonin reuptake inhibitors*. John Wiley; 1991.

(95) Shapira B, Reiss A, Kaiser N et al. Effect of imipramine treatment on the prolactin response to fenfluramine and placebo challenge in depressed patients *J Aff Dis* 1989; 16: 1–4.

(96) Corven PJ, Geaney DP, Schachter M et al. Desipramine treatment in normal subjects: effects of neuroendocrine responses to tryptophan and on platelet serotonin-related receptors. *Arch Gen Psychiat* 1986; 43: 61–7.

(97) Lesch KP, Hoh A, Schulte HM et al. Long term fluoxetine treatment decreases $5HT_{1a}$ receptor responsivity in obsessive-compulsive disorder. *Psychopharmacology* 1991; 105: 415–20.

(98) Manji HK, Hsiao JK, Risby ED et al. The mechanism of action of lithium. *Arch Gen Psychiat* 1991, 48: 505–12.

(99) Cowen PJ, McCance SL, Ware CJ et al. Lithium in tricyclic resistant depression. Correlation of increased brain 5HT function with clinical outcome. *Br J Psychiat* 1991; 159: 341–6.

(100) Shapira B, Lever B, Kindler S et al. Enhanced serotonergic responsivity following electroconvulsive therapy in patients with major depression. *Br J Psychiat* 1992; 160: 223–9.

(101) Mitchell PB, Bearn JA, Corn TH & Checkley SA. Growth hormone response to clonidine after recovery in patients with endogenous depression. *Br J Psychiat* 1988; 152: 34–8.

(102) Nurnberger JI, Berrettini W, Simmons-Alling S et al. Blunted ACTH and cortisol response to afternoon tryptophan infusion in euthymic bipolar patients. *Psychiat Res* 1990; 31: 57–67.

(103) Upadahyaya AK, Pennell I, Cowen PJ, Deakin JFW. Blunted growth hormone and prolactin responses to L-tryptophan in depression: a state dependent abnormality. *J Aff Dis* 1991; 21: 213–8.

(104) O'Keane V, O'Hanlon M, Webb M & Dinan T. D-fenfluramine/prolactin response throughout the menstrual cycle: evidence for an oestrogen-induced alteration. *Clin End* 1991; 34: 289–92.

(105) Marks MN, Wieck A, Checkley SA and Kumar R. Contribution of psychological and social factors to psychotic and non-psychotic relapse after childbirth in women with previous histories of affective disorder. *J Aff Dis* 1992; 29: 253–64.

(106) Greenstein B. Steroid hormone receptors in the brain. In: Lightman SL, Everitt BJ, Neuroendocrinology, Oxford; Blackwell Scientific Publications, 1986: 32–48.

(107) Koch M, Ehret G. Immunocytochemical localisation and quantitation of oestrogen-binding cells in the male and female (virgin, pregnant, lactating) mouse brain. *Brain Res* 1989; 489: 101–12.

(108) Sar M, Stumpf WE. Simultaneous localisation of 3H estradiol and neurophysin I or arginine vasopressin in hypothalamic neurons demonstrated by a combined technique of dry-mount autoradiography and immunohistochemistry. *Neurosci Letts* 1980; 17: 179–84.

(109) Bearn JA, Fairhall KM, Robinson ICAF et al. Changes in a proposed new neuroendocrine marker of oestrogen receptor function in postpartum women. *Psychological Med* 1990; 20: 779–83.

(110) Bearn JA, Lightman SL and Checkley SA. Estrogen receptor function in menopausal women. *Br J Clin Pharmacol* 1992. In press.

(111) Deakin JFW. Relevance of hormone–CNS interactions to psychological changes in the puerperium. In: Kumar R, Brockington IF eds. *Motherhood and mental illness 2*. London: Wright, 1988: 113–32.

(112) Clopton J, Gordon JH. In vivo effects of oestrogen and 2–hydroxyestradiol on D2 dopamine receptor agonist affinity states in rat striatum. *J Neural Trans* 1986; 66: 13–20.

(113) Gordon JH, Perry KD. Pre-and postsynaptic neurochemical alterations following oestrogen induced striatal dopamine hypo-and hypersensitivity. *Brain Res Bull* 1983; 10: 425–8.

(114) Wieck A, Kumar R, Hirst AD et al. Increased sensitivity of dopamine receptors

and recurrence of affective psychosis after childbirth. *Br Med J* 1991; 303: 613–6.

(115) Brockington IF, Kelly A, Hall P, Deakin W. Premenstrual relapse of puerperal psychosis. *J Aff Dis* 1988; 14: 287–92.

(116) Wieck A, Hirst AD, Kumar R et al. Growth hormone secretion by human females in response to apomorphine challenge is markedly affected by menstrual cycle phase. *Br J Clin Pharm* 1989; 27: 700–1P.

(117) McEwen BS, Coirini H, Westlind-Danielsson A et al. Steroid hormones as mediators of neural plasticity. *J Steroid Biochem Molec Biol* 1991; 39: 223–32.

(118) Meaney MJ, Viau V, Bhatnagar S, et al. Cellular mechanisms underlying the development and expression of individual differences in the hypothalamic-pituitary-adrenal stress response. *J Steroid Biochem Molec Biol* 1991; 39: 265–74.

(119) Matsumoto A. Synaptogenic action of sex steroids in developing and adult neuroendocrine brain. *Psychoneuroendocrinology* 1991; 16: 25–40.

(120) Diamond MC. Hormonal effects on the development of cerebral lateralization. *Psychoneuroendocrinology* 1991; 16: 121–9.

(121) Reinisch JM, Ziemba–Davis M, Sanders SA. Hormonal contributions to sexually dimorphic behavioral development in humans. *Psychoneuroendocrinology* 1991; 16: 213–78.

(122) Hampson E. Estrogen-related variations in human spatial and articulatory-motor skills. *Psychoneuroendocrinology* 1990; 15: 97–111.

(123) Gouchie C, Kimura D. The relationship between testosterone levels and cognitive ability patterns. *Psychoneuroendocrinology* 1991; 16: 323–34.

(124) Bachevalier J, Hagger C. Sex differences in the development of learning abilities in primates. *Psychoneuroendocrinology* 1991; 16: 177–88.

(125) Meaney MJ, Aitken DH, Sharma S, Viau V. Basal ACTH, corticosterone and corticosterone-binding globulin levels over the diurnal cycle, and age-related changes in hippocampal type I and type II corticosteroid receptor binding capacity in young and aged handled and nonhandled rats. *Neuroendocrinology* 1992; 55: 204–13.

From antibody to gene in schizophrenia: a review of the technology and a progress report

W G HONER and J L KENNEDY

Introduction

The pathogenesis and etiology of diseases of the nervous system are intimately related at the molecular level. Elucidating pathogenesis is important for the development of new therapeutic measures to alleviate the symptoms or alter the course of the illnesses. Knowledge of etiology may allow the development of preventative measures to decrease the incidence of certain diseases. The present paper describes a strategy developed to study both the mechanism and etiology of brain diseases in a parallel, synergistic fashion. The emphasis will be on the application of this approach to the investigation of schizophrenia.

To study the mechanism of illness in schizophrenia, we have focused on evaluating differences in brain proteins between cases of schizophrenia and controls. Since the brain proteins implicated in schizophrenia are largely unknown, a screening method was needed to identify proteins of potential interest. Techniques for separating and comparing different proteins have progressed steadily from the mid 1960s. Using gel electrophoresis, approximately 100–150 different protein bands could be resolved in brain tissues[1]. The development of two-dimensional gel electrophoresis increased this by an order of magnitude, to approximately 1500 different proteins[2]. Even with this power of resolution, success in defining molecular abnormalities in the brain in mental illness has been poor. However, improvement of another order of magnitude was achieved through the use of monoclonal antibody technology. With antibodies, proteins with relative abundance in the brain of 1 in 10 000 or less can be detected (P Davies, unpublished data).

All correspondence to: Dr W G Honer, Department of Psychiatry, University of British Columbia, Jack Bell Research Centre, 2660 Oak Street, Vancouver, BC, Canada V6K 3Z6.

Cambridge Medical Reviews: Neurobiology and Psychiatry Volume 2

Monoclonal antibodies can also be used to screen tissue samples to identify relevant proteins. The earliest applications of monoclonal antibody based screening in neurobiology were studies designed to define molecular differences between cell types in the nervous system[3,4]. Essentially, the antibodies allow 'molecular dissection' of tissue samples. Relatively crude brain homogenates from one tissue can be used to immunize mice. The spleen cells from these mice are then fused to mouse myeloma cells. The resulting hybrid cells can secrete monoclonal antibodies. The antibodies can be compared for selectivity of binding to the tissue used in the immunization versus binding to a second tissue; or antibody binding to specific cell types within one tissue can be studied. Once an antibody of interest is defined by some selective or differential binding property, the antibody can be used to isolate and purify the antigen. Characterization of the antigen will define a molecular difference between the tissues or cell types being investigated. The antigens defined may be already well-characterized molecules, or may be previously uncharacterized, novel molecules. This screening approach was used by Davies' group to develop monoclonal antibodies which showed relative differences in binding between control human brain tissue and tissue from cases of Alzheimer's disease[5]. The success of this approach in studies of Alzheimer's disease (AD) lead us to investigate the pathogenesis of schizophrenia using a similar methodology.

The second component of the strategy involves study of the etiology of schizophrenia, from a genetic perspective. Family, twin and adoption studies all indicate that there is a substantial genetic component to the etiology of the illness[6]. The advent of DNA-based genetic technology, combined with advances in the statistical evaluation of genetic inheritance has provided a powerful methodology for molecular studies of the genetic etiology of schizophrenia. Like the studies of mechanism, the studies of genetic etiology also require a screening technique. In this case, the genome must be screened to isolate and identify genes which predispose to the development of schizophrenia. One approach to accomplish this goal is to use anonymous genetic markers composed of restriction fragment length polymorphisms (RFLPs), or a new type of marker called a microsatellite repeat. The cosegregation of these markers with schizophrenia in multiplex families can be studied. Once a marker is found that cosegregates with schizophrenia, then efforts can proceed to identify the nearby gene which is related to the development of the illness.

Rather than searching with anonymous markers, a second approach is to directly target for study those genes which are potentially implicated in the mechanism of illness. This strategy is described as the candidate gene approach, and uses known genes to develop marker probes. The candidate gene approach links mechanism to etiology, and the present strategy is an extension of this. In our studies of etiology, the genes or gene segments chosen for linkage analysis are related to the proteins identified by monoclonal antibodies as being of interest in the pathogenesis of schizophrenia. As well as being used to characterize proteins, the antibodies serve as a bridge between the studies of etiology and mechanism. This is achieved by using the antibodies to screen expression vector libraries for cDNAs.

An expression vector library is an in vitro system which allows bacteria to express foreign proteins. To construct a human brain expression library, messenger RNA is first isolated from a sample of human brain tissue. The mRNA is then converted into the more stable cDNA form, and inserted into specially designed bacteriophage. Each bacteriophage generated carries a copy of a fragment of human cDNA which may code for a region of a brain protein. Bacteria are then infected with the phage, and under the appropriate induction conditions, the phage/bacterial system can synthesize or express the human brain protein segments coded for by the cDNAs. The same antibodies which identify proteins in brain tissue samples can then be used to isolate phage which carry cDNA fragments that code for a protein segment to which the antibody can bind. These antibody selected cDNA (AScDNA) fragments can then be developed into probes for linkage studies in schizophrenia pedigrees.

In order for an AScDNA to be useful as a linkage probe, several requirements must be met. First, a polymorphism in or near the functional gene must be visualized by the probe. Once a polymorphism can be detected, then the degree of cosegregation of the AScDNA and schizophrenia can be studied in multiplex pedigrees using genetic linkage analysis. Knowledge of the chromosomal assignment of the AScDNA, and the location of the AScDNA in the genetic map of the chromosome may be of value should there be a cluster of genes in the immediate region that could contribute to the illness. Genetic linkage analysis, and sequencing the gene in affected individuals are the ultimate tests of the relevance of the region identified by the AScDNA to the etiology of schizophrenia.

Methodological issues
A schematic diagram of the methodology of the antibody to gene approach appears in Fig. 1.

Developing antibodies for the study of schizophrenia
For this investigation, tissue was chosen from several limbic and other brain regions with putative neurochemical abnormalities in schizophrenia. The regions used were the nucleus accumbens, the caudate, the amygdala and the temporal and cingulate cortices. Pairs of mice were immunized with separate brain regions, and a total of 7600 hybridoma cell lines were generated. An enzyme linked immunoadsorbent assay (ELISA) method was used to screen

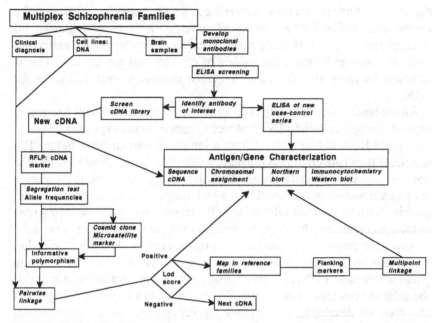

Fig. 1. Schematic illustrating the steps involved in the antibody to gene strategy for schizophrenia research. In this Figure, the brain samples used to generate the antibodies are illustrated as coming from the same families used in the genetic studies. This approach would maximize the sensitivity of the strategy, but has not yet been attempted by us.

the hybridoma cell lines for those producing antibodies of interest: defined as those showing differential binding to pooled schizophrenia versus pooled control brain homogenates. Following studies of the pooled samples, the cell lines producing antibodies worthy of further investigation were cloned. The individual samples of schizophrenia and control brain homogenates were then studied using each of the antibodies in a fully quantitative assay. These results were used to select antibodies for further studies involving antigen characterization.

Antigen characterization Three approaches were used to characterize the antigens identified as being of potential relevance to studies of schizophrenia. Additional quantitative ELISA studies were carried out with homogenates to determine the regional brain distribution of the antigens, and to indicate if the antigens were brain specific. Immunocytochemical studies were carried out using formalin fixed human brain tissue to determine the cellular distribution of the antigens. This information also complemented the quantitative ELISA studies of regional brain distribution. Finally, the molecular weight of the antigens was studied using SDS-polyacrylamide gel electrophoresis and Western blotting techniques.

Antibody selected cDNAs The studies of antigen characterization indicated that the antigen reactive with antibody EP10 was of most interest. To isolate cDNAs coding for a segment of protein with an EP10 binding site, the antibody was used to screen a human temporal cortex cDNA library (Clontech) in λgt11 (2×10^6 plaque forming units). Preliminary characterization of the AScDNAs isolated was carried out by determining the length of each insert using agarose gel electrophoresis.

Developing a linkage probe, and preliminary linkage studies One of the AScDNAs isolated (clone WH4) was further characterized. To test for an RFLP, the cDNA was labelled by nick translation for hybridization to a polyscreen containing DNA samples from ten unrelated individuals, digested with a set of 20 restriction enzymes. As well, the DNA sequence of WH4 was determined and compared to the sequences available in the Genbank database. To determine the chromosomal assignment of the clone, the sequence information was used to generate two primers for polymerase chain reaction (PCR). The primers were used in a PCR screen of a human-hamster hybrid cell panel. Each hybrid cell line contained human DNA from a known subset of human chromosomes, and PCR product was generated only from those cell hybrids containing the chromosome on which WH4 was localized. Finally, once the chromosomal assignment was established, the RFLPs were used to perform linkage mapping in reference families. This established the position of the WH4 clone in the genetic linkage map, and determined the allele frequency of the RFLPs. This information complemented the chromosomal assignment results and was needed for linkage studies of schizophrenia. In collaboration with other investigators, preliminary linkage results were generated for Italian and Swedish families with schizophrenia, using the RFLPs for the WH4 probe.

Antibodies of interest for the study of schizophrenia

Studies of brain homogenates pooled separately from cases of schizophrenia and from controls indicated that 19 cell lines were producing an antibody of interest. Seventeen of these cell lines were successfully cloned and the antibodies produced were designated the EP series. Antibodies from 12 of these hybridomas were subsequently reported to show selectivity for schizophrenia or control tissues in a small pilot study[7].

Antigen characterization Partial characterization of the antigens implicated a variety of molecules as possibly contributing to the pathophysiology of schizophrenia (see Table 1 and Fig. 2). The antigen recognized by antibody

Table 1. *Description of the EP series of antibodies developed through immunization of mice with schizophrenia brain tissue*

Antibody	ELISA	ICC	WB	Notes
EP1	+	+	–	Neuronal cell body and dendritic staining, also reactive with red blood cells
EP2	+	+	–	Neuronal cell body and dendritic staining, also reactive with red blood cells
EP6	+	+	+	Diffuse grey matter staining, apparent molecular weight 45 kD, brain specific
EP7	+	+	–	Cell process staining, especially in cortex, also reactive with lymphocytes
EP8	+	+	–	Fine fibre-like meshwork, especially white matter, also reactive with lymphocytes
EP9,13,14	+	+	–	Fine fibre-like meshwork, especially white matter, brain specific
EP10	+	+	+	Synaptic vesicle related protein, apparent molecular weight 38 kD
EP11	+	+	–	Diffuse staining, brain specific
EP15	+	+	–	Diffuse grey matter staining, limited reactivity with liver
EP16	+	+	–	Astrocytic staining, also reactive with liver
EP17	+	+	–	Fine fibre-like meshwork, especially white matter, limited reactivity with lymphocytes
EP19	+	+	–	Fine fibre-like meshwork, especially white matter, brain specific

ICC: immunocytochemistry, WB: Western blot. The antigens are not completely characterized in most cases for this series of antibodies. Antibodies were tested by ELISA for reactivity with brain, lung, liver, red blood cell and lymphocyte homogenates, and with serum.

EP10 was characterized in most detail[8]. As demonstrated by immunocyctochemistry, the EP10 antigen was localized to grey matter. The pattern of distribution of the antigen in the cerebellum was compatible with a presynaptic localization. Western blotting studies (Fig. 3(a)) indicated that the molecular weight of the antigen was approximately 38 000 daltons, and immunoprecipitation studies using an antibody against the synaptic vesicle protein synaptophysin indicated that the EP10 antigen was synaptophysin-like.

An EP10 AScDNA Five cDNA clones were isolated from the temporal cortex library after screening with EP10. Each was 370–385 base pairs in length, and likely represent multiple copies of the same mRNA, although this was not studied definitively. The clone designated WH4 was studied further.

Developing a linkage probe from the AScDNA

Clone WH4 was found to be 381 base pairs in length. Earlier searches of DNA databases indicated that the clone did not have significant sequence homology with known genes. However, a search of the most recent release of the Genbank database reveals a significant sequence homology between WH4 and the human gene for the integrin α_3 subunit. The clone detects two RFLPs in genomic DNA (Fig. 3(b)) digested with the restriction enzymes BglII and MspI[9]. In the somatic cell hybrid study, PCR product was generated from primers derived from WH4 only in hybrid cell lines containing human chromosome 17 (Fig. 4). WH4 was then assigned the locus D17S444E, and the RFLPs were used to perform linkage mapping in reference pedigrees. These studies indicated that D17S444E is tightly linked (lod score > 11) to two other loci of interest in neurobiology, the homeobox-2 gene cluster (HOX2@) and nerve growth factor receptor (NGFR) (see Fig. 5). Both of these loci are involved in the development of the nervous system, HOX2@ in controlling aspects of segmentation, and the NGFR gene product in the development of cholinergic neurons.

Preliminary linkage studies The RFLPs for WH4 were used to test for linkage to schizophrenia in a large Swedish kindred segregating schizophrenia, and in several smaller Italian families. Assuming a single major locus model, autosomal dominant transmission, penetrance = 0.70, disease gene frequency = 0.0085 and phenocopies = 0.001, the lod scores were significantly negative. These results imply that under the model specified the D17S444E locus is not linked to schizophrenia in these families[10,11].

The antibody to gene strategy described for the study of schizophrenia originated from basic neurobiological research. Each component of the strategy depends on one or more assumptions, which form a context for the interpretation of the results. These factors will be discussed, focusing

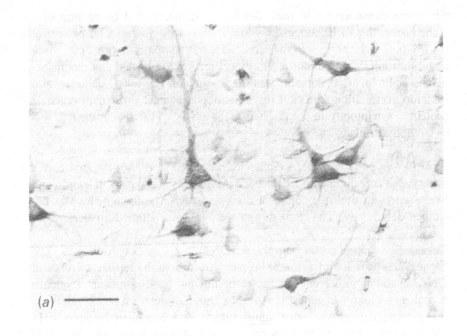

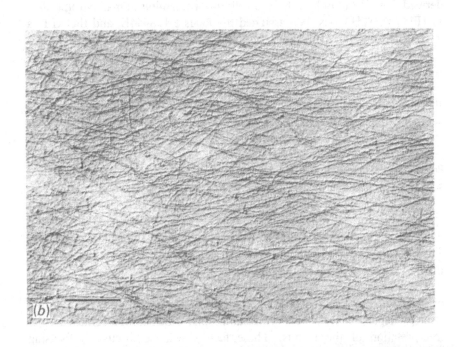

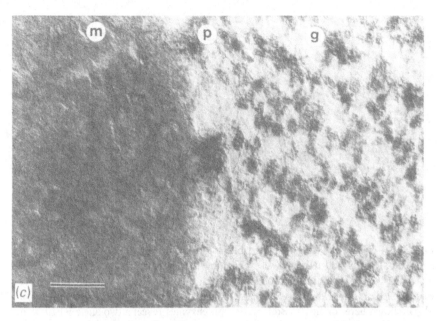

Fig. 2. (*a*) Staining of neuronal cell bodies and proximal dendrites in cingulate cortex with antibody EP2. EP1 staining was similar. Bar represents 50 μ. (*b*) Staining of cellular processes in CA1 region of hippocampus with antibody EP7. Bar represents 50 μ. (*c*) Staining of the cerebellum with antibody EP10. Diffuse staining was observed in the molecular layer (m), focal staining was seen in the Purkinje cell (p) and granule cell (g) layers, and no staining was seen in the white matter (not shown). This pattern is typical of that seen with antibodies directed against molecules located in the presynaptic compartment. Bar represents 50 μ.

primarily on the antibody component of the strategy since the methodological issues concerning genetic linkage in schizophrenia are well described elsewhere[12,13]. While the present paper is primarily oriented towards presentation of the strategy, a brief consideration of the preliminary results will follow this.

Antibody component

Assumptions The possibility of developing schizophrenia selective monoclonal antibodies relies on several assumptions. First, the antigen or antigens relevant to the disease process must be present in the tissue used for immunization. Choice of tissue therefore requires some knowledge of the sites and mechanism of pathology in schizophrenia. Although significant brain tissue destruction does not occur in this illness, the antigens of interest could still be absent or markedly reduced in the tissues chosen for immuniza-

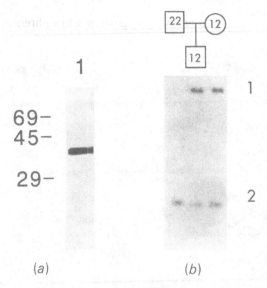

(a)   (b)

Fig. 3. (a) Immunoblotting (Western blot) study of the EP10 antigen. The band at approximately 38 000 daltons was stained by the EP10 antibody. The position of molecular weight standards in kilodaltons is indicated on the left. (b) The probe WH4 was labelled and hybridized to Southern blotted DNA samples digested with enzyme MspI (shown here) or BglII. Both restriction enzymes reveal a two-allele RFLP that was useful as a DNA marker for genetic linkage studies.

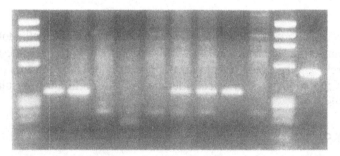

Fig. 4. PCR of the WH4 site in human, chimp and BIOS™ hybrid cell panel DNAs. An initial hypothesis was that the WH4 sequence might be part of a known synaptic gene cluster on the X chromosome. However, hybrid cell panel DNAs containing the X chromosome revealed no PCR product. The PCR reaction revealed product only in those hybrid cell DNAs containing chromosome 17 (other panel DNAs not shown). In order to confirm the identity of the PCR product, restriction digests were done with two enzymes, BanII and NcoI. The digestions showed restriction fragments of the expected sizes.

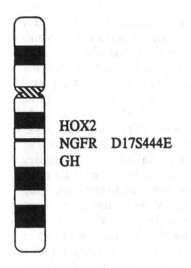

HOX2
NGFR **D17S444E**
GH

17

Fig. 5. Chromosome 17 ideogram with the standard 'G' banding pattern. The probe WH4 detects MspI and BglII RFLPs. These polymorphisms were used to map the locus recognized by WH4 to the 17q21–22 region, very close to the HOX2@ gene cluster, and to the gene for nerve growth factor receptor. Lod scores for this location are >11 in pairwise genetic linkage analyses.

tion. Should this be the case, a strategy of immunizing with control tissue and screening the antibodies generated could be successful. Similarly, if a significant component of schizophrenia is developmental in origin, the antigens initially responsible for the illness may be expressed only transiently. In this case, the contribution of studying the tissues at postmortem may be to identify secondary changes in other antigens which could provide clues to the proximate molecular lesion. A final caveat is that the antigen in question must be immunogenic.

Criteria defining a useful antibody Mice will generate large numbers of antibodies after immunization with human brain, and the primary limiting factor in screening for antibodies of interest is often the endurance of the investigator. Criteria for deciding which antibodies to pursue intensively are required in order to optimize the investment of time and resources into screening based studies. The following criteria are suggested:

1. The antibody defines a quantitative or qualitative difference between the diseased and control tissues.
2. The antibody is useful in various assay formats. Quantitative assays

such as an ELISA may be needed to define differences between control and disease states. Qualitative assays such as immunocytochemistry and Western blotting are important in characterizing the disease related antigen identified by the antibody. Finally, an antibody of maximal versatility will also be useful in isolating cDNAs coding for the antigen.

3. The antibody defines an interesting antigen. As Sutcliffe[14] has pointed out, there are likely to be between 30 000 and 50 000 genes selectively expressed in the brain, and the protein products of only a small fraction of these are known. Screening strategies allow a degree of serendipity to come into play, and although the optimum antibody may be elusive, many interesting antibodies can be developed along the way. Of note, antibodies developed for the study of brain molecules in one illness may be equally, or even more useful in the study of other brain diseases not included in the screening scheme. This was the case for several of the antibodies developed by Davies' group for the investigation of AD; a subset of these antibodies was equally interesting for the study of Pick's disease[5,15,16]. Similarly, several of the EP series have proven of value in studies of AD[17] and of epilepsy (Honer et al., in preparation).

Tissues for immunization In the present study, the diseased tissues were used for immunization. Screening was carried out through comparison of antibody binding to diseased versus control tissues. The anatomical regions chosen were based on those suspected at the time to contain neurochemical abnormalities in schizophrenia. Other interesting antibodies might be developed by immunizing with control tissues. Using the latter approach, an antibody raised against normal human spinal cord identified heterotopic spinal cord neurons in patients with amyotrophic lateral sclerosis[18,19]. A further possibility is to test panels of antibodies raised against neural tissues from other species. In one application of this approach, an antibody developed against cholinergic synaptosomes from the *Torpedo* ray exhibited reduced binding to AD tissue sections compared to controls[20,21]. In a different series of studies, several antibodies developed through immunizations with *Drosophila* heads showed relatively increased or decreased binding to AD brain tissues[22,23].

A further consideration is preparation of the tissue prior to immunization. The immunizations for the EP series were performed using tissue homogenates. Other investigators studying animal brain have had less success using raw homogenates, and suggest the use of various enrichment procedures prior to immunization[24]. These include physical methods such as ultracentrifugation, or chromatography using lectin or antibody columns. Others suggest removing highly immunogenic molecules from tissue extracts prior to immunization[25]. The present approach of using raw homogenates likely maximizes the range of antigens presented to the immune system. The strategy suggested to increase the yield of useful antibodies is to immunize with raw brain homogenate; then increase the power of the screening methods to focus on the most versatile antibodies produced.

Immunization protocols

As part of the genesis of an immune response, antigens are processed into short peptide fragments by the immune system. These short peptides contain epitopes or binding sites complementary to the antigen binding sites of antibodies. The timing and frequency of immunizations will influence the affinity of the antibodies produced, the range of antibody subclasses generated, and the range of epitopes detected. In general, cell fusions performed after regular immunizations over a period of months will generate high affinity antibodies, predominantly IgG molecules directed against a limited series of dominant epitopes. In contrast, cell fusions performed after only one or two immunizations will produce low as well as high affinity antibodies, including more IgM molecules, and the range of epitopes detected will be larger. For screening studies where a number of fusions are necessary, testing antibodies from both short and long immunization protocols may be advantageous.

New protocols are suggested to use the animal's immune system to advantage in suppressing the production of antibodies equally reactive with reference and target tissues. The neonatal tolerization and the cyclophosphamide suppression strategies involve conditioning the immune system through immunization with the reference tissue, suppressing or deleting the clones of antibodies produced, then reimmunizing with the target tissue[26,27]. The goal is to increase the yield of antibodies selective for the target tissue. These approaches could be used in attempting to develop schizophrenia selective antibodies through immunizing initially with control tissue, then using schizophrenia tissue as the challenge. The strategy might also work with the order of immunizations reversed. Although these and other completely novel approaches[28] to generating antibodies hold promise, the screening strategy adopted for antibody selection remains critically important.

Screening methodology

A broad range of antibodies are generated after immunization with human brain tissue, reactive with a wide variety of processed antigens. These antibodies will detect brain antigens in screening assays, provided the epitopes to which they bind are not distorted or destroyed due to tissue processing. As well as preservation of epitopes, the design of a screening assay must take several other considerations into account. Screening a large number of hybridomas will increase the possibility of isolating an antibody of interest. Obtaining the maximum amount of information regarding the versatility of the antibody as early as possible, even prior to cloning the hybridoma line, can prevent wasting effort on suboptimal antibodies. The methods available for screening include immunocytochemistry, Western blotting and ELISA.

The inherent characteristics of each assay determine the amount of information revealed regarding the usefulness of the antibody.

Most neurobiology investigations involving panels of monoclonal antibodies have used immunocytochemistry as a screening assay. The principal advantage of this method is the large amount of information revealed about the antigen detected. The distribution of the antigen will be apparent, and with experience interpreting immunocytochemistry, hypotheses can quickly be developed regarding the nature of the antigen as well as the elements of the nervous system expressing the molecule. These features are optimum for basic science studies, where relatively few hybridomas (perhaps hundreds) may need to be screened before focusing on several antibodies of interest.

Immunocytochemistry is somewhat limited as a screening technique for human brain studies. The first problem is that of numbers. For schizophrenia studies, several thousand antibodies may require screening and immunocytochemistry is quite labour intensive. A second problem concerns heterogeneity within the illness. Immunocytochemical methods require comparison of tissue from single control individuals to single diseased individuals, thus reducing the sensitivity of the screening technique unless massive numbers of sections are stained. This is not a problem in basic science research where individual differences between healthy, often inbred animals are likely to be minimal. For schizophrenia studies, immunocytochemistry may be a useful screening technique if the goal is to develop antibodies identifying a feature of the illness such as heterotopic neurons in the entorhinal cortex[29,30] and if the number of antibodies screen can be minimized through techniques such as neonatal suppression.

If Western blotting could be used as a screening technique, a large amount of highly important information regarding differences in antigens between disease and control brains would be immediately available. This would be especially true if 2-dimensional gels were used. However, this approach is relatively impractical for screening thousands of hybridoma supernatants, and has the additional disadvantage of difficulties in quantifying results.

Semiquantitative solid phase assays were the screening method of choice for the present studies. In these assays, control and schizophrenia brain homogenates were dried onto 96 well microplates. The homogenates were pooled from several individual brains, and applied at a standardized protein concentration. The hybridoma supernatants were applied in duplicate to wells containing control brain homogenate, and to wells containing schizophrenia brain homogenate. The development of a microplate assay using peroxidase-coupled secondary antibodies enabled large numbers of hybridoma supernatants to be assayed in a semiautomated fashion. This is the major advantage of the ELISA as a screening technique. If homogenates of known protein concentration are premade, a single operator can perform all of the steps for screening 500 or more hybridoma supernatants per day using the ELISA method. Other investigators have used a similar screening technique but with nitrocellulose as a solid phase ('dot blot' assay)[31].

The ELISA methodology does have several limitations. Protein structure is altered by binding to the ELISA plate, and epitopes may become distorted or unavailable for antibody binding[32,33]. To limit nonspecific binding, blocking solutions are used prior to the incubation of samples with antibody. Differences in blocking solutions appear to influence the ability to detect antigen–antibody interactions. The present experience indicates that 5% powdered, nonfat milk in buffered saline provides a more complete suppression of nonspecific binding than bovine serum albumin (and is significantly less costly). However, the possibility does exist that some specific binding is also inhibited by the blocking step, and relevant antibody binding may be missed as a consequence. The most useful antibodies are those that are reactive with samples in more than one assay format. Antibodies which detect brain molecules in an ELISA may not be useful for immunocytochemistry or Western blotting. Similarly, an antibody selected on the basis of an immunocytochemical screen may not be useful for the development of a quantitative assay based on an ELISA. For those antibodies which do detect antigen in the ELISA assay, a final consideration is the sensitivity of the assay in comparing the amount of antigen present in samples of control and diseased brain homogenates. As configured for the present studies, the assay aims to have the amount of antigen as the limiting feature, with excess concentrations of both the primary and secondary antibodies. This increases the sensitivity of the assay, however, if a relatively abundant antigen differs between disease and controls, the assay may not detect this due to saturating conditions. A more likely possibility is that the antigens of interest may be rare, and the number of antibody molecules bound to the antigen immobilized on the ELISA plate may be below the detection threshold of the assay. New technical developments in substrates and detection instruments may increase the sensitivity of these immunoassays.

A recent study used the ELISA technique as a screening method to detect antibodies developed after immunization with a synaptic vesicle associated immunoprecipitate[34]. To increase the information yield prior to cloning the hybridomas, micromethods were used to test the ELISA positive hybridoma supernatants with immunocytochemistry. The cerebellum was chosen as a target tissue for immunocytochemistry since several synaptic antigens have a characteristic distribution there. Small fragments were cut from Vibratome sections of formalin fixed tissue, and incubated with aliquots of hybridoma supernatants using 96 well microplates. Hybridomas were only cloned if the antibody produced was useful in both assays. This sequential screening approach could be modified and incorporated into studies designed to screen for schizophrenia selective antibodies.

W G Honer and J L Kennedy

Statistical considerations

The design of studies involving screening small numbers of cases and controls
with large numbers of antibodies raises interesting questions regarding the
role of statistics and probability in determining the experimental outcome.
The first consideration is defining how many tests are actually being performed. Thousands of hybridoma supernatants may be tested. However,
studying 10 000 hybridoma cells does not imply that 10 000 distinct
monoclonal antibodies are being assessed, nor does it imply that 10 000
distinct antigens are being assayed. The following factors need to be considered. First, only a portion of the hybridoma cells generated may actually
be secreting antibody, others may have lost this capacity. Secondly, many
hybridomas may be producing antibodies against the same antigen. Thirdly,
as described previously, the screening assay will have the potential to yield a
positive result with only a subset of the antibodies produced due to technical
limitations. In the EP series, only 14% of the hybridomas screened were
secreting detectable antibody against brain antigens.

Even if the number of possible positive results is in the thousands rather
than the tens of thousands, a reasonably large number of antibodies ought to
show differences between samples from control and diseased brains by
chance alone. However, this assumes that at the screening stage completely
quantitative measures are made on individual samples from the two populations studied, using each antibody, and that the mean results are compared.
This is not actually the case. In practice, a small number of samples of
diseased brains are pooled, assayed and the results compared to those
obtained from a small number of samples from control brains. In the screening stage, the assay is performed at a single protein concentration. Antibody–antigen interactions are kinetically similar to enzyme–substrate
interactions, and the single point measure obtained in the screening assay is
only an estimate of the actual antigen concentration. An arbitrary value of a
difference in optical density measurement of approximately 2-fold is used to
identify antibodies for further study. It is likely that differences in antigen
concentration between groups must be 2-fold or greater to be detected in the
screening assay. Whether or not this difference in antigen concentration
between the groups is due to chance operating through the variability in the
antigen within each population, or due to the illness cannot be determined
definitively through studying the same samples used to screen for antibodies
of interest. If there is a large difference between cases and controls, and a
small degree of variability within the control population in the amount of the
antigen present, then it is more likely that the result represents the effects of
illness rather than chance. A more definitive conclusion requires testing the
antibody in a different group of cases and controls to determine if a statistically significant difference in the amount of antigen detected exists. This
remains to be determined for the EP antibodies in schizophrenia. However,

the broader objective of developing interesting antibodies was achieved for the EP series, as several of these antibodies identify antigens of neurobiologic interest, and do show differences in binding between AD and control brains[8,17].

Statistical considerations regarding antibody screening studies are complex, since the number of distinct assays actually being performed is unclear, the variability within the population being studied is unknown, the assay is probably insensitive to differences smaller than 2-fold, and the same difference in signal between samples may represent a difference in antigen concentration of 2-fold to 30-fold for different antigens. Based on empiric experience, a reasonable approach may be to select antibodies based on an optical density difference of at least 0.3 when pooled samples are compared, then proceed to test the individual samples. If the difference is confirmed in a quantitative study using dilution curve analysis, and there is minimal overlap between individual case and control samples, then testing the antibody in a new, larger series of cases and controls would appear to be indicated.

Genetic component

If schizophrenia selective antibodies can be developed with the technology described, then the protein sequence of the antigen defined by the antibody could be used to clone a gene of potential etiologic importance in schizophrenia. This is the traditional candidate gene approach. Rather than fully defining genes based on protein sequence data, the present proposal is to use the antibodies to directly isolate AScDNAs, which can be used as linkage probes. There are merits as well as pitfalls in this proposal.

All genetic linkage methods seek cosegregation of the illness with a gene marker. If anonymous RFLPs are used, multitudes of markers may need to be screened before linkage is found. One proposed improvement is to use cDNAs as markers[35]. Since these are expressed sites, the probability of finding linkage using cDNA markers may be increased relative to the use of anonymous probes. AScDNAs may offer an additional opportunity to increase the yield of linkage studies, particularly if part of the selection process involves the use of antibodies which are disease selective. However, the relationship between the AScDNA and the brain antigen detected by the antibody may not be straightforward.

Monoclonal antibodies bind to short segments of protein, which may be only 4–6 amino acids in length[36]. In screening a cDNA library with a monoclonal antibody, the possibility exists that the fusion protein detected may share nothing but a small region of homology or other similarity with the brain protein detected by the antibody in tissue samples. The likelihood is high that more than one clone will be detected through antibody screening of expression vector libraries. However, knowing the precise relationship between the AScDNA and the brain protein may not be necessary for genetic screening studies. The development of panels or families of AScDNAs may serve to increase the sensitivity of the genetic screen. Recent work in the genetics of muscular dystrophy provides an interesting example relevant to this possibility. Duchenne muscular dystrophy is due to an abnormality of the X chromosome gene coding for the dystrophin protein. Lien et al.[37] hypothesized that related genes could be involved in other forms of muscular dystrophy. They identified an antibody against the C-terminus of dystrophin as having cross reactivity with another protein, then used the antibody to isolate a cDNA which was characterized as coding for microtubule-associated protein 1B (MAP-1B). This cDNA did not have any primary DNA or predicted amino acid sequence homology to dystrophin. Like dystrophin, however, MAP-1B is a cytoskeletal related protein. The MAP-1B cDNA was localized to chromosome 5q, and was found to be tightly linked to the locus for spinal muscular atrophy, a different form of muscular dystrophy.

A final possible advantage of the AScDNA approach is that even if the gene identified is not a direct etiological factor in schizophrenia, the causative pathway in the brain may be revealed through examination of nearby genes implicated through linkage. This possibility is enhanced by a tendency for genes of related function to cluster within the genome, as in the example of the haemoglobin genes.

Progress report

The pathogenesis and etiology of schizophrenia remain unclear. Data from the antibody to gene project indicate several areas of possible focus. Characterization of the EP10 antigen as a synaptic vesicle related protein suggests that study of synapses in schizophrenia through analysis of their molecular constituents may be of value. This approach would complement the traditional neuropharmacological approach to the illness. Others have also suggested the potential importance of synaptic mechanisms to the pathogenesis of schizophrenia, and place these into a neurodevelopmental context[38].

The AScDNA clone WH4 was found to have significant sequence homology with one of the integrin subunit genes. This could be a false positive finding, since the relationship of the antibody binding fusion protein to the native brain antigen has not yet been clarified. Integrins are receptor molecules for extracellular matrix proteins such as cell adhesion molecules[39]. Integrins are not yet described as having a role in synaptic vesicle function, however it is of interest that integrins are reported to be packaged as part of neutrophil cell granules[40]. Integrins are also involved in neural development. The WH4 clone was localized to a region of chromosome 17 in close proximity to two other loci involved in neural development, HOX2i and NGFR. The preliminary linkage data reported here do not support a role for this region of the genome in the etiology of schizophrenia, assuming a single major locus model. Heterogeneity within schizophrenia may be a factor complicating the results. Ideally, the brain tissue used to develop the antibodies for the project would come from the same pedigrees or at least the same populations as those being tested for linkage. This was not the case in the first application of the approach, where the brain tissues used were obtained from Washington, DC, and the pedigrees tested were from Italy and Sweden. We are continuing to test WH4, using pedigrees from different ethnic populations as well as statistical techniques which model interacting loci[41].

In summary, the results indicate that the antibody to gene strategy outlined is technically feasible. Repeated attempts will be necessary to localize genes of etiological importance to schizophrenia. However, progress from the antibody to gene approach will also be derived through the development of monoclonal antibodies and gene markers of value for studies of the pathogenesis and etiology of other human brain disorders. We are optimistic about the future prospects of this moderately comprehensive, synergistic strategy for schizophrenia research.

Acknowledgement

This work was supported by the National Alliance for Research on Schizophrenia and Depression, the Canadian Psychiatric Research Foundation, and the British Columbia Health Research Foundation. Drs Anne Bassett and Peter Davies provided helpful advice during the development of the ideas presented in this paper.

References

(1) Moore BW, McGregor D. Chromatographic and electrophoretic fractionation of soluble proteins of brain and liver. *J Biol Chem* 1965; 240: 1647–53.

(2) O'Farrell PH. High resolution two-dimensional electrophoresis of proteins. *J Biol Chem* 1975; 250: 4007–21.

(3) Barnstable CJ. Monoclonal antibodies which recognize different cell types in the rat retina. *Nature* 1980; 286: 231–5.

(4) Zipser B, McKay R. Monoclonal antibodies distinguish identifiable neurones in the leech. *Nature* 1981; 289: 549–54.

(5) Wolozin BL, Pruchnicki A, Dickson DW, Davies P. A neuronal antigen in the brains of Alzheimer patients. *Science* 1986; 232: 648–50.

(6) Gottesman II, Shields J. *Schizophrenia: the epigenetic puzzle*. Cambridge: Cambridge University Press, 1982.

(7) Honer WG, Kaufmann CA, Kleinman JE, Casanova MF, Davies P. Monoclonal antibodies to investigate the brain in schizophrenia. *Brain Res* 1989; 500: 379–83.

(8) Honer WG, Kaufmann CA, Davies P. Characterization of a synaptic antigen of interest in neuropsychiatric illness. *Biol Psychiat* 1992; 31: 147–58.

(9) Kennedy JL, Honer WG, Kaufmann CA, Martignetti JA, Brosius J, Kidd KK. Two RFLPs near HOX2@/NGFR at locus D17S444E. *Nucleic Acids Res* 1992; 20: 1171.

W G Honer and J L Kennedy

(10) Kennedy JL, Honer WG, Gelernter J et al. New candidate genes for schizophrenia. *Schizophr Res* 1991; 4: 280.

(11) Kennedy JL, Honer WG, Martignetti J et al. Antibody selection for candidate genes in schizophrenia-linkage studies. *Psychiat Gene* 1991; 2: 31–32.

(12) Kennedy JL, Giuffra LA. Recent developments in genetic linkage studies of schizophrenia. In: Schultz C, Tamminga C, eds. *Schizophrenia research.* New York: Raven Press, 1991.

(13) Weeks DE, Brzustowicz L, Squires-Wheeler E et al. Report of a workshop on genetic linkage studies in schizophrenia. *Schizophrenia Bull* 1990; 16: 673–86.

(14) Sutcliffe JG. mRNA in the mammalian central nervous system. *Ann Rev Neurosci* 1988; 11: 157–98.

(15) Scicutella A, Davies P. Marked loss of cerebral galactolipids in Pick's disease. *Ann Neurol* 1987; 22: 606–9.

(16) Scicutella A, Davies P. Characterization of monoclonal antibodies to galactolipids and uses in studies of dementia. *J Neuropathol Exp Neurol* 1988; 47: 406–19.

(17) Honer WG, Dickson DW, Gleeson J, Davies P. Regional synaptic pathology in Alzheimer's disease. *Neurobiol Aging* 1992; 13: 375–82.

(18) Hinton DR, Henderson VW, Blanks JC, Rudnicka M, Miller CA. Monoclonal antibodies react with neuronal subpopulations in the human nervous system. *J Comp Neurol* 1988; 267: 398–408.

(19) Kozlowski MA, Williams C, Hinton DR, Miller CA. Heterotopic neurons in spinal cord of patients with ALS. *Neurology 1989; 39: 644–8.*

(20) Kushner PD. A library of monoclonal antibodies to *Torpedo* cholinergic synaptosomes. *J Neurochem* 1984; 43: 775–86.

(21) Kushner PD, Stephenson DT, Wright S, Cole GM, Greco CM. Monoclonal antibody *Tor* 23 binds a subset of neural cells in the human cortex and displays an altered binding distribution in Alzheimer's disease. *J Neuropathol Exp Neurol* 1989; 48: 692–708.

(22) Fujita SC, Zipursky SL, Benzer SL, Ferrus A, Shotwell SL. Monoclonal antibodies against the *Drosophila* nervous system. *Proc Nat Acad Sci USA* 1982; 79: 7929–33.

(23) Miller CA, Rudnicka M, Hinton DR, Blanks JC, Kozlowski M. Monoclonal antibody identification of subpopulations of cerebral cortical neurons affected in Alzheimer's disease. *Proc Nat Acad Sci USA* 1987; 84: 8657–61.

(24) Schlosshauer B, Wild M. Generation of monoclonal antibodies specific for developmentally regulated antigens of the chicken retina. *Dev Brain Res* 1991; 59: 197–208.

(25) Woodhams PL, Webb M, Atkinson DJ, Seeley PJ. A monoclonal antibody, Py, distinguishes different classes of hippocampal neurons. *J Neurosci* 1989; 9: 2170–81.

(26) Hockfield S. A Mab to a unique cerebellar neuron generated by immunosuppression and rapid immunization. *Science* 1987; 237: 67–70.

(27) Matthew WD, Sandrock AW. Cyclophosphamide treatment used to manipulate the immune response for the production of monoclonal antibodies. *J Immunol Meth* 1987; 100: 73–82.

(28) Winter G, Milstein C. Man-made antibodies. *Nature* 1991; 349: 293–9.

(29) Jakob H, Beckmann H. Prenatal developmental disturbances in the limbic allocortex in schizophrenics. *J Neural Transm* 1986; 65: 303–26.

(30) Falkai P, Bogerts B. Qualitative and quantitative assessment of pre-alpha-cell clusters in the entorhinal cortex of schizophrenics. A neurodevelopmental model of schizophrenia? *Schizophr Res* 1991; 4: 357–8.

(31) Hawkes R, Niday E, Matus A. Monoclonal antibodies identify novel neural antigens. *Proc Nat Acad Sci USA* 1982; 79: 2410–14.

(32) Mierendorf RC, Dimond RL. Functional heterogeneity of monoclonal antibodies obtained using different screening assays. *Anal Biochem* 1983; 135: 221–9.

(33) Wognum AW, Lansdorp PM, Eaves CJ, Krystal G. Use of a sensitive bioimmunoabsorbent assay to isolate and characterize monoclonal antibodies to biologically active human erythropoietin. *Blood* 1988; 71: 1731–7.

(34) Honer WG, Hu L, Davies P. Human synaptic proteins with a heterogeneous distribution in cerebellum and visual cortex. *Brain Res* 1993; in press.

(35) McKusick VA. Current trends in mapping human genes. *FASEB J* 1991; 5: 12–20.

(36) Fieser TM, Tainer JA, Geysen M, Houghten RA, Lerner RA. Influence of protein flexibility and peptide conformation on reactivity of monoclonal antipeptide antibodies with a protein α-helix. *Proc Nat Acad Sci USA* 1987; 84: 8568–72.

(37) Lien LL, Boyce FM, Kleyn P et al. Mapping of human microtubule-associated protein 1B in proximity to the spinal muscular atrophy locus at 5q13. *Proc Nat Acad Sci USA* 1991; 88: 7873–6.

(38) Feinberg I. Schizophrenia: caused by a fault in programmed synaptic elimination during adolescence? *J Psychiat Res* 1982–83; 17: 319–34.

(39) Reichardt LF, Tomaselli KJ. Extracellular matrix molecules and their receptors: functions in neural development. *Ann Rev Neurosci* 1991; 14: 531–70.

(40) Bainton DF, Miller LJ, Kishimoto TK, Springer TA. Leukocyte adhesion receptors are stored in peroxidase-negative granules of human neutrophils. *J Exp Med* 1987; 166: 1641–53.

(41) Vieland V, Greenberg DA, Hodge SE, Ott J. Linkage analysis of two-locus diseases under single-locus and two-locus analysis models. *Cytogenet Cell Genet* 1992; 59: 145–6.

Neurotrophins and neurodegenerative disease

D DAWBARN, S J ALLEN and S H MacGOWAN

Background

Neurodegenerative diseases are characterized by the selective degeneration of discrete neuronal nuclei. Parkinson's disease, for example, is known to involve a loss of neurons in the substantia nigra, the symptoms of amylotrophic lateral sclerosis are associated with the degeneration of motor neurons and in Alzheimer's disease (AD) the cholinergic neurons of the basal forebrain are particularly vulnerable. It is generally assumed that it is the loss of neocortical cholinergic function (often measured as a reduction in neocortical choline acetyltranferase activity; ChAT) which is responsible for the cognitive deficits in AD although other neurons are also known to be affected. It has been assumed that for each neuronal system there must be specific proteins released by the target issues which act as survival factors. These proteins have been termed neurotrophic factors and it is hoped that they can be used pharmacologically for the treatment of neurodegenerative disease.

The first discovered neurotrophic protein was β-nerve growth factor (β-NGF) which was identified in a mouse sarcoma[1]. Subsequent studies showed that the male mouse submaxillary gland contains relatively large amounts which enabled the purification and sequencing of the protein. β-NGF exists as a homodimer with a molecular weight of 26 000 Da and a pI of 9.3.

The physiology of β-NGF in the peripheral nervous system is well understood and it has been shown to act as a neurotrophic factor for sympathetic and sensory neurons[2]. More recently β-NGF and its mRNA have been detected in the central nervous system where the content was shown to correlate with the degree of basal forebrain cholinergic innervation suggesting that β-NGF may act as a neurotrophic factor for these cholinergic neurons[3].

All correspondence to: Dr D Dawbarn, Molecular Neurobiology Group, Department of Medicine (Care of the Elderly), University of Bristol, Bristol Royal Infirmary, Bristol BS2 8HW, UK

Cambridge Medical Reviews: Neurobiology and Psychiatry Volume 2
© Cambridge University Press

Distribution of β-NGF receptors in the brain

Receptor autoradiographic studies have shown β-NGF receptors to be localized on rodent basal forebrain neurons[4,5]. It has been shown that injection of [^{125}I]β-NGF into the rodent hippocampus results in the accumulation of radioactivity in the neurons of the medial septal nucleus and the diagonal band of Broca (dbB), cholinergic basal forebrain neurons which are known to project to the hippocampus[6]. We and others have confirmed the localization of the low affinity β-NGF receptor (p75[NGFR]) to rodent basal forebrain neurons using a monoclonal antibody (IgG192)[7-9]. In addition, by staining alternate sections through the rat basal forebrain with antibodies to p75[NGFR] and to ChAT, a marker for cholinergic neurons, we have shown that the majority of basal forebrain cholinergic neurons express the low affinity receptor[10].

Using a monoclonal antibody raised against human p75[NGFR] (ME20.4), we have examined the distribution in human brain[11]. Staining was only observed in neurons and was punctate in appearance, perinuclear staining was often observed as was staining of dendrites and axons (Fig. 1). The distribution of immunoreactive neurons was followed in a caudal direction from their appearance in the septum until their disappearance at the level of the substantia nigra (Fig. 2). This followed closely the distribution of the hyperchromic magnocellular neurons of the basal forebrain which has previously been described in human brain[12-14]. Immunopositive neurons were observed rostrally at the medial edge of the lateral ventricle in the dorsal and medial septal nuclei. At the level of the globus pallidus and the preoptic area, and in sections immediately caudal to this, two distinct groups of neurons were present in the dbB, one medial and the other positioned laterally. Numbers of neurons increased caudally. At the level of the emergence of the anterior commissure, only the ventral aspect of the dbB remained, caudally merging with more lateral neurons to form the anterior portion of the nucleus basalis (NBCh4a). Large numbers of immunoreactive neurons were observed in the intermediate portion of the nucleus basalis (NBCh4i) at the level of the ansa peduncularis, which can often be seen to divide NBCh4i into dorsal and ventral groups. At the level of the descending limb of the anterior commissure three main groups of neurons formed the posterior portion of the nucleus basalis (NBCh4p). These lay between the dorsal edge of the descending limb of the anterior commissure and the optic tract. In each brain examined the neurons seen most caudally were those ventral to and extending into the external medullary lamina at the level of the substantia nigra. In addition to these main groups of neurons other smaller surrounding groups were observed throughout the length of the dbB and NBCh4. In addition, immunoreactive neurons were occasionally seen embedded in the white matter of the anterior commissure and more frequently in the fibre tracts of the ansa peduncularis and the ansa lenticularis. Four normal brains were

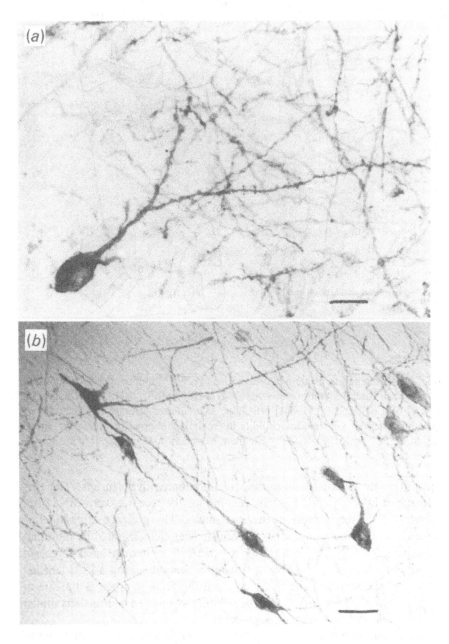

Fig. 1. High power photomicrographs of neurons, immunoreactive for p75^{NGFR}, from the NBCh4 region of a normal human brain. Scale bars are (a) 50 μm, (b) 100 μm.

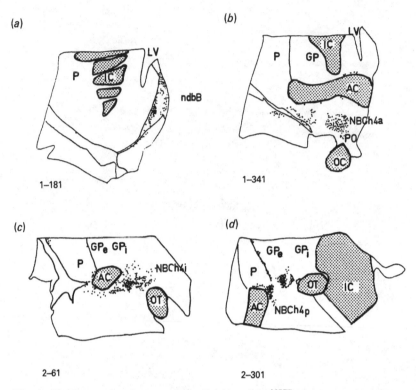

Fig. 2. Representative diagram of distribution of p75[NGFR] immunopositive neurons in four human basal forebrain sections from (a) [1–181] ndbB, (b) [1–341] NBCh4a, (c) [2–61] NBCh4i, and (d) [2–301] NBCh4p. AC: anterior commissure; GP$_e$: globus pallidus external; GP$_i$: globus pallidus internal; IC: internal capsule; LV: lateral ventricle; OC: optic chiasm; OT: optic tract; P: putamen; PO: preoptic area.

quantitatively assessed for numbers of immunoreactive neurons. The percentage of hyperchromic neurons staining for the receptor were 78%, 82%, 85% and 91% respectively in the four nuclei. The presence of cholinergic neurons in the human brain has previously been demonstrated by immunocytochemistry[15–18]. The localization of p75[NGFR] to human basal forebrain membranes was confirmed by in situ hybridization[11] using a [^{35}S] labelled cDNA probe which also established basal forebrain neurons as the site of synthesis of p75[NGFR] (Fig. 3). The distribution of labelled neurons was similar to that observed by immunocytochemistry.

Administration of β-NGF to rodent cholinergic neurons both in vitro and in vivo has been shown to increase cholinergic function as measured by an increase in ChAT activity[19–24]. Fimbria–fornix lesions in rodents sever the connections between the hippocampus and the cholinergic medial septal neurons and result in retrograde degeneration of these septal neurons. This

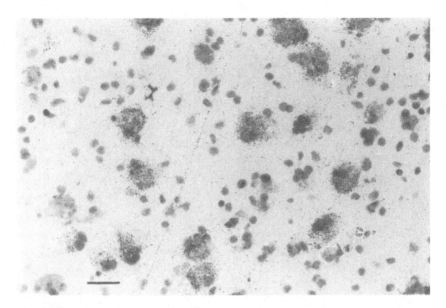

Fig. 3. High power photomicrograph of basal forebrain magnocellular neurons following in situ hybridization with [^{35}S]-labelled cDNA probe for p75^{NGFR}. Positive neurons are identified by deposits of silver grains. Sections are counter-stained with haemotoxylin. X200. Scale bar is 50 μm.

degeneration can be completely reversed by administration of NGF into the cerebrospinal fluid using miniosmotic pumps[25–28]. Similar results have also been obtained in primates following fimbria–fornix lesions[29,30]. Administration of NGF has also been shown to reverse spatial memory learning deficits in rats with basal forebrain lesions[31] and in aged rats[32].

Patients suffering with AD have severe memory impairments which have been associated with an observed reduction in ChAT activity[33]. Since β-NGF has been shown to increase ChAT activity and reverse memory defects in rodents, as detailed above, it has been widely suggested that administration of β-NGF to AD patients may be therapeutic. For β-NGF to be of benefit, it has been assumed that there should be sufficient functional β-NGF receptors present on surviving cholinergic basal forebrain neurons.

Comparison of β-NGF receptors in normal and AD brain

Using the antibody ME20.4 we have compared the number and size of neurons expressing p75^{NGFR} in different subdivisions of the basal forebrain in normal brain and in AD (Fig. 4)[34]. In some patients, there was a reduction in the number of neurons in one or more subdivisions, although no region was more likely to be affected than any other. In the majority of sections of AD

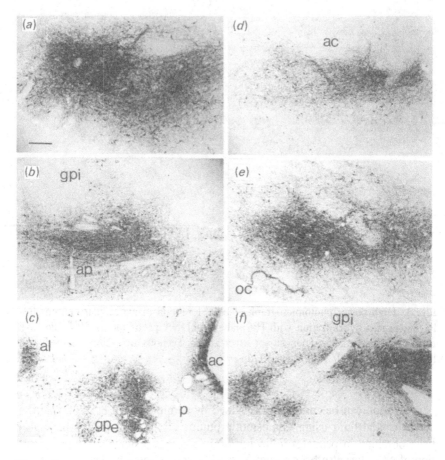

Fig. 4. Low power photomicrographs of human basal forebrain sections stained with anti-p75^{NGFR} antibodies. (*a*), (*b*) and (*c*) normal; (*d*), (*e*) and (*f*) AD. (*a*) and (*d*) NBCh4am; (*b*) and (*e*) NBCh4i; (*c*) and (*f*) NBCh4p. Scale bar is 500 μm.

brain examined there were many surviving immunoreactive neurons. In one AD patient, with only 9% of normal neocortical ChAT activity, there was still 40% of neurons remaining overall in the NBCh4 region. The number of neurons counted in three areas of the NBCh4 region in AD was between 66% and 72% of normal mean values (Fig. 5), although due to the variation between patients there was no statistically significant reduction in number of neurons in any region of the ndbB or NBCh4 compared with normal data. Two other studies have, by contrast, reported a more marked neuronal loss[35,36]. These two studies, respectively, report a loss of 61% and 62.5% of neurons in the NBCh4 region in AD compared with normal. This is most

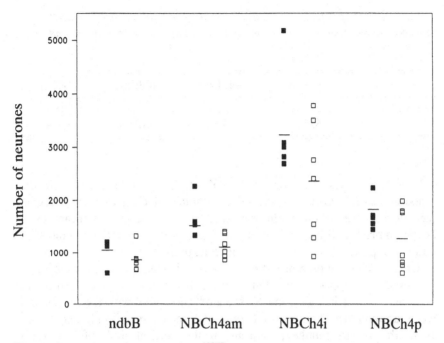

Fig. 5. Comparison of number of p75^NGFR immunopositive neurons in four sections from five normal [■] and seven AD [□] basal forebrain.

likely to be related to the younger mean age of their AD subjects; those AD patients most affected in our study, not only in terms of neuronal loss but also in tests of cognitive function and ChAT activity, were also the youngest. Statistical analysis of pooled AD data revealed an increase in percentage of proportion of small neurons in the ndbB, NBCh4am and NBCh4i with a decrease in larger neurons. This change became more obvious when individual cases were examined for neuronal size distribution.

We found no change in percentage of hyperchromic magnocellular neurons which were β-NGF receptor immunoreactive in those regions of the basal nuclei with a reduced number of neurons (Table 1). This suggested that it was not only the β-NGF receptor positive neurons which were affected, which is in accord with the qualitative observations of others[37] who found no 'decoupling' of the colocalization between β-NGF receptor and ChAT immunoreactivity. In normal and AD basal forebrain they found that most neurons appeared to stain with antibodies against both the receptor and ChAT. It is quite possible then, that there is not a large reduction in expression of receptors, although it will be necessary to quantify numbers of receptors or the level of receptor mRNA per neuron before one can be sure.

D Dawbarn et al

Table 1. *Immunopositive neurons as a percentage of total number of hyperchromic magnocellular neurons in four regions of the basal nucleus in five normal and seven AD brains*

	ndbbB	NBCh4am	NBCh4i	NBCh4p
Normal	71±10	79±6	79±7	90±4
AD	67±7	72±3	81±7	85±4

In AD, a marked reduction of ChAT activity has been reported in the hippocampus[33,38]. Characteristic neuropathological changes in this region seem to occur early on in the disease. Since the human hippocampus is known to produce β-NGF[39] it is curious that there was no reduction found in number of β-NGF receptor positive neurons in the ndbB in our study of AD patients, despite the presence of numerous senile plaques and neurofibrillary tangles in the hippocampus. This study supports an earlier assessment of neuronal number in AD using Nissl stain[40] and agrees with the results of a recent immunohistochemical study of β-NGF receptors[36]. If in human brain, as in the rhesus monkey, neurons in the vertical limb of the ndbB predominantly project to the hippocampus and hypothalamus, then early changes in the hippocampus would be expected to affect neurons of the ndbB. The ndbB however, appears to be the least affected region of the basal forebrain in AD.

ChAT activity was found to correlate with number of neurons in all areas of the NBCh4 region examined demonstrating that the extent of neuronal loss was related to cortical cholinergic function (Fig. 6). The lack of correlation seen between number of neurons in the ndbB and occipital ChAT activity may be explained by the fact that there are few projections between the ndbB and the occipital cortex, as observed in the rhesus monkey[41].

Using a cDNA probe to p75[NGFR] we have examined the distribution p75[NGFR] mRNA in normal brain by Northern analysis[42]. A single 3.7 kb band was seen in striatum, thalamus, hippocampus and cerebellum although the highest levels were seen in basal forebrain extracts. A comparison of the content of basal forebrain p75[NGFR] mRNA from five patients who had died with no neurological symptoms and from five who had died with a histologically confirmed diagnosis of AD showed no difference although cortical ChAT activity was considerably reduced (Fig. 7).

We have examined the binding characteristics of [I[125]]-2.5S NGF to membrane preparations from basal forebrain samples[43]. Tissue samples were homogenized in buffered 0.32 M sucrose with a Janssen ultra-turrax (30s, 4 °C) and centrifuged (10 min at 7700 g, 4 °C) to remove cell debris. The supernatant was recentrifuged (60 min 100 000 g, 4 °C) to pellet membranes

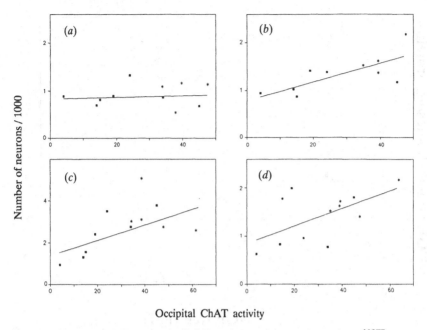

Fig. 6. Correlation of occipital ChAT activity with number of p75^{NGFR} positive neurons counted in four sections in [*] normal and [■] AD subjects in (a) ndbB (b) NBCh4am (r=0.63) (c) NBCh4i (r=0.59) and (d) NBCh4p (r=0.59). Correlation coefficients of (b), (c) and (d) are significant at $p \leqslant 0.05$.

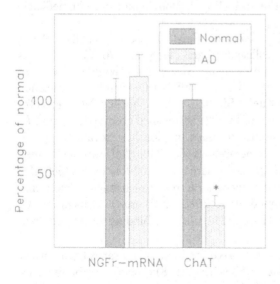

Fig. 7. Levels of p75^{NGFR} mRNA in five normal and five AD basal forebrains compared with temporal ChAT activity. ChAT activity was reduced to 29% of normal value compared with no significant change in p75^{NGFR} mRNA.

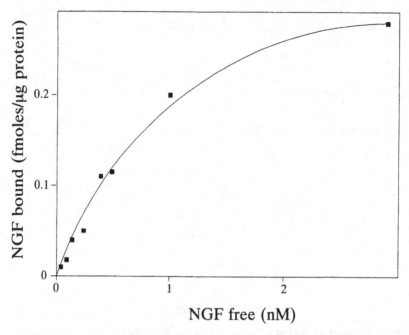

Fig. 8. Saturation curve of [^{125}I]-2.5S NGF binding in basal forebrain membranes from a normal brain.

which were resuspended in 100 mM PBS, aliquoted and frozen immediately at −70 °C.

2.5S NGF was purified from 100 pairs of male mouse submaxillary glands as described by Mobley and colleagues[44] and stored at −70 °C. Purity was checked against commercial samples using SDS-polyacrylamide gel electrophoresis and isoelectric focusing. NGF was radiolabelled using a modification of the lactoperoxidase technique[45]. Binding of radiolabelled NGF to A875 cells, PC12 cells and membranes of PC12 (unpublished observations) gave K_d or B_{max} values which were similar to those previously reported[46,47]. [^{125}I]-NGF binding to basal forebrain membranes (60–350 μg/ml) was determined (20 pM–6 nM), specific binding was displaced by a 100-fold excess (600 nM) of unlabelled 2.5S NGF. Each point was the result of triplicate determinations. Binding data was analysed using Enzfitter (Biosoft). Cytochrome C, insulin and epidermal growth factor did not displace binding when used up to the μM range.

Steady-state saturation analysis of basal forebrain membranes from normal and AD brain with radiolabelled 2.5S NGF (Fig. 8) revealed one binding site which corresponded to the low affinity size previously reported in other species[48,49]. There was no significant difference in mean K_d or B_{max} between normal and AD brain tissue (Fig. 9). The mean K_d values ± sem for normal

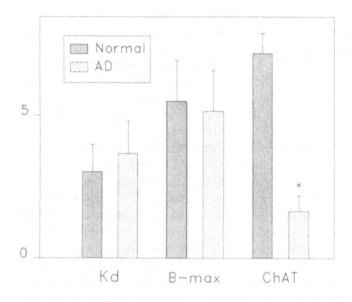

Fig. 9. Binding of $[^{125}I]$-2.5S NGF to its receptor in basal forebrain membrane preparations from five normal and five AD brains. Kd (nM), Bmax (fmol X 10 $[^{125}I]$-2.5S NGF bound/1 μg membrane protein) and parietal ChAT activity (pmol acetyl-choline produced/100 μg protein/min). Values are mean ± sem.

and AD basal forebrain membranes were 3.02 nM ± 0.93 and 3.67 nM ± 1.16, the mean B_{max} values were 0.55 ± 0.14 and 0.52 ± 0.15 fmoles/μg membrane protein. By contrast, mean ChAT values were significantly redu-ced ($p \geqslant 0.001$) in AD. Receptor binding studies in intact PC12 cells and cell membranes (unpublished observations) revealed two binding sites which corresponded to the high and low affinity binding sites. In membranes prepared from human basal forebrain, only the low affinity receptor was detectable.

β-NGF content in normal and AD brain
In aged rat brain a 40% reduction of β-NGF in the hippocampus has been reported[50]. Since β-NGF acts as a trophic factor for basal forebrain cholinergic neurons, it has been speculated that the reduction in cholinergic function in AD may be caused by a loss of β-NGF in the cortex and hippocampus.

We have used a modification of a sensitive and specific two site ELISA[51,52] to measure the content of β-NGF in AD brain[53]. Four cortical regions and the hippocampus were examined in brains obtained at autopsy from AD patients and intellectually unimpaired subjects. ChAT activity was measured in the temporal cortex, Brodmann area (BA) 21, from the same brains. Anti-β-NGF antibody (clone 27/21, Boerhinger; 50 µl of 0.4 µg/ml in coating buffer: 50 mM NaCO$_3$ pH 9.6) was pipetted onto washed microtitre plates and left overnight at room temperature. Nonspecific sites were then blocked with buffer containing 1% BSA for two hours at room temperature. Microtitre plates were washed (wash buffer: 50 mM Tris HCl pH 7.0, 200 mM NaCl, 0.05% sodium azide, 0.25% gelatin and 0.1% Triton X-100) using a Nunc microtitre plate washer. Brain tissue was sonicated (sonic probe, 5 × 60 seconds) in extraction buffer (2X wash buffer excluding Triton X-100 containing 2% BSA, 4 mM EDTA, 40 U/ml aprotinin, 0.2 mM phenylmethylsulphonyl fluoride in dimethylsulphoxide, 0.2 mM benzethonium chloride and 2 mM benzamidine). Homogenates were subsequently centrifuged at 15 000 g for 30 minutes at 10 °C. Supernatants were diluted 1:1 (v/v) with 0.2% Triton X-100. Standards (mouse β-NGF, Boerhinger) were in the range of 10 pg/ml to 1 ng/ml. Samples and standards (50 µl) were pipetted into microtitre wells and incubated overnight at room temperature. Microtitre plates were washed and incubated for 2 hours at 37 °C with anti-β-NGF-galactosidase (clone 27/21; Boerhinger, 50 µl of 100 mU/ml in wash buffer containing 1% BSA). Finally, after su..equent washing, substrate solution (50 µl) was added. The substrate 4-methyl-umbelliferyl-β-D galactoside (substrate buffer: 100 mM sodium phosphate pH 7.3 containing 1 mM MgCl$_2$ and 0.1% sodium azide) produced a fluorescent product which could be measured using a fluorometer (Fluoroskan II: excitation wavelength 355 nm, emission wavelength 460 nm).

Normal cortical β-NGF levels were (mean ± sem) 408 ± 77, 459 ± 48, 264 ± 43 and 221 ± 32 pg/g wet weight in BA21 (medial temporal gyrus), BA22 (superior temporal gyrus), BA10 (frontal cortex) and BA7a (parietal cortex) respectively. Normal hippocampal β-NGF levels were 1396 ± 407 pg/g wet weight which is much higher than that found in the cerebral cortex. This is comparable to the relative amounts found in the rat brain. β-NGF content was not significantly different from normal levels in the same regions taken from AD brain (Fig. 10). ChAT activity measured in BA21 was reduced by at least 85% in each AD patient compared with normal. Postmortem delay and β-NGF content did not correlate in any of the brain regions examined.

Our data show that the loss of ChAT activity in AD neocortex and hippocampus, areas in which AD neuropathology is most readily apparent, is not due to a reduction in β-NGF content. The antibody that was used in this study was initially raised against 2.5S mouse NGF, although it has been shown by several groups that it is able to cross-react with recombinant human β-NGF. Biological activity of the recombinant β-NGF has also been shown to be consistent with the amount detected by the antibody[54].

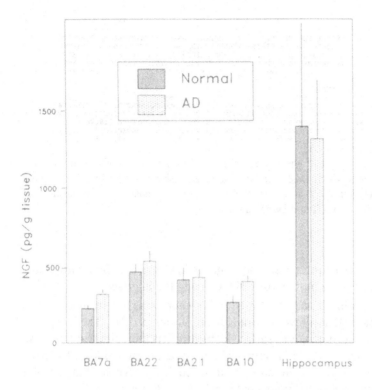

Fig. 10. β-NGF content in normal and AD hippocampus and parietal (BA7a), temporal (BA22 and BA21) and frontal (BA10) cortex using a two-site ELISA.

Neurotrophins

In addition to the cloning of β-NGF[55-58], three other neurotrophic factor genes have been cloned which show considerable homology to β-NGF. Brain derived neurotrophic factor (BDNF)[59-61], neurotrophin-3 (NT-3)[61-65] and neurotrophin-4 (NT-4, sometimes called NT-5)[66-68] are all very basic proteins of approximately the same size with the six cysteine residues being absolutely conserved. Examination of the sequences reveals four variable domains (Fig. 11). Since the proteins have differing distributions and biological specificities it would seem appropriate to speculate that the variable domains are involved in conferring this specificity. The crystal structure of 2.5S NGF has been determined at a resolution of 2.3 Å although no electron density was observed for residues 1–10 (the amino terminus) and 112–118 (the carboxy terminus)[69]. Each monomer was shown to consist of seven β strands which contribute to 3 antiparallel pairs of β strands. In the β-NGF dimer two promoters assembled along a 2-fold axis with their long axis roughly parallel and their flat faces in

131

D Dawbarn et al

```
                         I                                    II
Human NGF    --SSSHPIFHRGEFSVCDSVSVWVG--DKTTATDIKGKEVMVLGEVNINNS-VFKQYFFETKC
Human BDNF   --HSDPA--RRGELSVCDSISEWVTAADKKTAVDMSGGTVTVLEKVPVSKG-QLKQYFYETKC
Human NT3    --YAEHKS-HRGEYSVCDSESLWVT--DKSSAIDIRGHQVTVLGEIKTGNS-PVKQYFYETRC
Human NT4    GVSETAPASRRGELAVCDAVSGWVT--DRRTAVDLRGREVEVLGEVPAAGGSPLRQYFFETRC
              .*** .***. * **   *. .* *. *  * **  .    .  .***.**.*

                       III                          IV
Human NGF    RD-------PNPVDSGCRGIDSKHWNSYCTTTHTFVKALTMDG-KQAAWRFIRIDTACVCVLSRKAVRRA
Human BDNF   NP-------MGYTKEGCRGIDKRHWNSQCRTTQSYVRALTMDSKKRIGWRFIRIDTSCVCTLTIKRGR--
Human NT3    KE-------ARPVKNGCRGIDDKHWNSQCKTSQTYVRALTSENNKLVGWRIRIDTSCVCALSRK-IGRT
Human NT4    KADNAEEGGPGAGGGGCRGVDRRHWVSECKAKQSYVRALTADAQGRVGWRIRIDTACVCTLLSRTG-RA
              ****.* .** * * . ...*.***  .  .** *****.*** *  .
```

Fig. 11. A comparison of the amino acid sequence alignment of human β-NGF, BDNF, NT-3 and NT-4. Dashes indicate gaps, asterisks show absolute conservation of amino acids, full stops show conservative amino acid changes. The positions of variable domains I, II, III and IV are shown.

contact at the dimer interface. The dimer is held together by hydrophobic forces derived from a number of residues along the interface.

Variable domains II and IV of β-NGF both appear as β-hairpin loops and variable domain III as a reverse turn (Fig. 12, facing p. 181). The identification of the variable domains as surface loops supports the claim that it is these regions which are involved in receptor binding particularly since it has been shown that surface β-hairpin loops are involved in the receptor binding of a wide range of proteins including epidermal growth factor[70].

trk receptors

In addition to the p75[NGFR] there is also a higher affinity receptor which binds β-NGF with a K_d of approximately 10^{-11} M. On primary sensory neurons[48] and β-NGF responsive cell lines, such as the rat pheochromocytoma cell line PC12[71,72], the high affinity receptor accounts for about 10% of the total number of β-NGF receptors. The higher affinity receptor also has a much slower rate of dissociation than p75[NGFR] and a greatly increased resistance to the action of proteolytic enzymes.

Cross linking experiments using [^{125}I] 2.5S mouse NGF showed that the high affinity receptor had a molecular weight of about 140 000 Da[73,74] and that the ligand receptor complex could be precipitated with antibodies to phosphotyrosine indicating that the receptor had tyrosine kinase activity. In 1986 Martin-Zanca and colleagues[75] isolated a human oncogene, tropomyosin receptor kinase (trk) from a colon carcinoma that was formed by the fusion of truncated tropomyosin and protein-tyrosine kinase sequences. The tyrosine kinase sequence was used to screen human cDNA libraries and the normal cellular counterpart of the oncogene, the trk proto-oncogene (referred to as trkA) was identified as a protein with an open reading frame of 790 amino acids with a molecular weight of 140 000 Da after glycosylation and referred

132

to as $p140^{trkA}$ [76]. Further screening of cDNA libraries using the tyrosine kinase sequences revealed the presence of two homologous proto-oncogenes trkB[77-79] and trkC[80] whose tyrosine kinase domains are 87% homologous at the amino acid level.

Northern analysis using probes for trkA, trkB and trkC showed that their expression was restricted to the nervous system[76,77,79,80]. This information together with the known size of the high affinity β-NGF receptor and the fact that it can be precipitated with anti-phosphotyrosine antibodies suggested that $p140^{trkA}$ may be the high affinity β-NGF receptor[74]. Several studies rapidly confirmed this hypothesis by showing that NGF binds to $p140^{trkA}$ with high affinity and that physiological concentrations of NGF also induce tyrosine phosphorylation of $p140^{trkA}$ in a rapid specific fashion affirming a method of signal transduction for β-NGF through $p140^{trkA}$ [81-84]. Subsequent studies showed that $p145^{trkB}$ can act as a receptor for BDNF, NT-3 and NT-4 but not NGF[68,85-88]. NT-3 has also been shown to act as a ligand for $p145^{trkC}$

We have examined the distribution of $p145^{trkB}$ in rat brain using various radiolabelled cDNA probes. Rat trkB (gift from Regeneron) was used to produce a 2988 bp probe coding for the entire cDNA to trkB; an 1100 bp probe coding only for the extracellular region by PCR and a 645 bp probe made from a Stu I/PstI fragment of the PCR probe. Subcloning of the extracellular PCR product into M13 produced both sense (M13 mp19) and antisense (M13 mp18) cDNA probes. Labelling was by random priming (Stratagene–Prime It) using ^{35}S-dATP (1300 Ci/mmol). Probes were purified using push columns (Stratagene–Nuctrap push columns). Sections were cryostat cut (20 µm) and dried onto poly-L-lysine covered slides. These were fixed in 4% buffered paraformaldehyde for five minutes, washed in PBS, then 70% ethanol and stored in 95% ethanol. All solutions were made with DEPC-treated water. All glassware was baked to inactivate contaminating RNase. Sections were hybridized in hybridization buffer (50% formamide, 5 × SSC, 50 mM sodium phosphate pH 7.0, 250 µm/ml heparin, 0.1% SDS, 10% dextran sulphate, 20 mM dithiothreitol) containing denatured ^{35}S-cDNA probe (150 000 cpm/20 µl buffer) and left overnight at 42 °C. Sections were subsequently washed three times at room temperature with 2 × SSC and overnight gently shaking at room temperature in 50% formamide, 0.6 M NaCl, 10 mM Tris hydrochloride buffer pH 7.4, 1 mM EDTA, 20 mM dithiothreitol. These were finally rinsed in 2 × SSC and dehydrated in 75% and then 95% ethanol. Sections were either laid on HyperS or β-Max (Amersham) autoradiography paper and exposed for a week or dipped in LM-1 emulsion (Amersham) and left to expose for 4–6 weeks.

Specific labelling was seen with all antisense probes. No labelling was seen with the sense probe. Particularly intense labelling was seen in the primary olfactory cortex and at the edge of the lateral ventricles, the third ventricle and the actuate hypothalamic nucleus. All layers, except layer I, of the

D Dawbarn et al

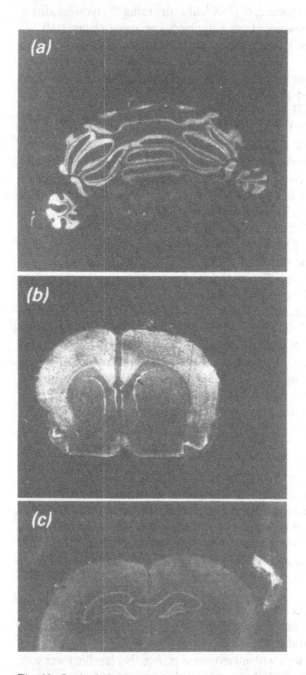

Fig. 13. In situ hybridization in A: cerebellum; B: forebrain, and C: hippocampus of 20 μm sections of rat brain using an 1100 base pair PCR amplified [^{35}S] cDNA probe for *trk*B.

134

cerebral cortex were labelled. Heavy labelling was also apparent in the pyramidal cells of Ammon's horn and the dentate gyrus of the hippocampus and in some layers of the cerebellum. Staining was apparent in several other nuclei including the cholinergic neurones of the basal forebrain (Fig. 13). The preliminary distributions of $p140^{trkA}$ and $p145^{trkC}$ have also been reported by other groups[80,89].

Therapeutic implications of neurotrophins

The suggestion that NGF could be used therapeutically in AD has largely been based on the identification of $p75^{NGFR}$ on basal forebrain cholinergic neurons and the effects of NGF on these neurons. It is still not known if these effects are mediated through $p75^{NGFR}$ or $p140^{trkA}$. It has been shown that NGF can mediate meiotic maturation of xenopus oocytes and is mitogenic to NIH 3T3 cells following transfection of each cell type with $trkA$[90,91]. In addition it has been shown that in mouse β-NGF mutation of lysines 32 and 34 to alanines in combination with the mutation of glutamic acid 35 to alanine completely abolishes binding to $p75^{NGFR}$ with only a small reduction in binding to $p140^{trkA}$. This analogue still induces neurite outgrowth in PC12 cells supporting the argument that biological activity is mediated through $p140^{trkA}$ [92].

In contrast, it has been shown that transfection of the gene encoding $p75^{NGFR}$ into mutant cells which do not express this protein restores high affinity binding and NGF induced protein phosphorylation suggesting that $p75^{NGFR}$ is involved in signal transduction[93–95]. It has also been shown that $p75^{NGFR}$ binds the other neurotrophins with equal affinity indicating that it may act as a common subunit for the other neurotrophin receptors[64,66,85,96,97]. Recently, mice have been generated which carry a mutation in the gene encoding $p75^{NGFR}$ by targeted mutation in embryonic stem cells[98]. Such animals showed defects in neuropeptide-containing sensory fibre innervation of peripheral tissues and concomitant reduction in sensitivity to heat stimulus. This behavioral abnormality can be ameliorated by crossing the mutant animals with another transgene encoding human $p75^{NGFR}$. It has also been shown that the maturational change that occurs in chick embryonic sensory neurons grown in vitro is retarded by the addition of antisense oligonucleotides to $p75^{NGFR}$ which prevent the expression of this receptor[99].

It would seem that both $p140^{trkA}$ and $p75^{NGFR}$ are required for biological activity. In relation to the therapeutic effects of NGF it would be illuminating to determine the distribution of $p140^{trkA}$ in human brain and in particular to determine whether or not basal forebrain cholinergic neurons express $p140^{trkA}$ in normal brain and also in AD. The distribution of $p145^{trkB}$ and $p145^{trkC}$ within the human nervous system should help to determine which neurons respond to BDNF, NT-3 and NT-4. This information can then be used to identify specific neurodegenerative diseases which can be targeted for treatment with neurotrophic proteins.

It has been shown that, in addition to NGF, BDNF can also increase ChAT activity of basal forebrain cholinergic neurons[100]. Although the content of β-NGF[53] and β-NGFmRNA[39] have been shown not to be reduced in AD brain one recent study has shown that BDNF mRNA is reduced in the hippocampus of AD brains[101] indicating that BDNF may be involved in the etiology of AD and may therefore be used therapeutically. One clinical study has looked at the effects of infusing mouse 2.5S NGF into the ventricles of a patient suffering from AD[102]. A total of 6.6 mg of 2.5S NGF was delivered over 3 months at a rate of 15 μl/hour corresponding to 75 μg/24 hours. The patient showed a marked increase in uptake and binding of ^{11}C-nicotine in frontal cortex interpreted as an increase in the density of cholinergic terminals. Cortical blood flow was also increased as measured by PET. After one month of treatment tests of verbal episodic memory were improved although other cognitive tests were not. The results from this study indicate that further trials with recombinant human β-NGF and BDNF are warranted in AD.

It has also been shown that, in addition to its effects on basal forebrain cholinergic neurons, BDNF can enhance the survival of mesencephalic dopaminergic neurons in culture and protect them from the neurotoxic effects of MPP$^+$ (1-methyl-4-phenylpyridinium; the active metabolite of MPTP, 1-methyl-4-phenyl-1,2,3,6-tetrahydropyridine)[103]. BDNF has also been shown to increase dopamine uptake of mesencephalic dopaminergic neurons[104]. These studies suggest that BDNF may have neurotrophic effects for dopaminergic neurons of the substantia nigra, neurons which are known to degenerate in Parkinson's disease. Further studies will be required to confirm these reports which if substantiated would indicate that clinical trials with BDNF in Parkinson's disease would be worthwhile.

In summary, it would appear that the treatment of neurodegenerative diseases using neurotrophins is still at an early stage although recent results indicate that these proteins may prove effective in combating these debilitating diseases.

Acknowledgements

This work was supported by the Medical Research Council, the Wellcome Trust, Bristol Research into Alzheimer's Disease and Care of the Elderly (BRACE), the Sandoz Foundation for Gerontological Research and the Halley Stuart Trust.

References

(1) Levi-Montalcini R. The nerve growth factor thirty-five years later. *EMBO J* 1987; 6: 1145–54.

136

(2) Thoenen H, Barde Y-A. Physiology of nerve growth factor. *Physiol Rev* 1980; 60: 1284–335.

(3) Korsching S, Auberger G, Heumann R, Scott J, Thoenen H. Levels of nerve growth factor and its mRNA in the central nervous system correlate with cholinergic innervation. *EMBO J* 1985; 4: 1389–94.

(4) Richardson PM, Verge Issa VMK, Riopelle RJ. Distribution of neuronal receptors for nerve growth factor in the rat. *J Neurosci* 1986; 6: 2312–22.

(5) Raivich G, Kreutzberg GW. The localization and distribution of high affinity β-nerve growth factor binding sites in the central nervous system of the adult rat. A light microscopic autoradiographic study using [^{125}I]-β-nerve growth factor. *Neuroscience* 1987; 20: 23–6.

(6) Seiler M, Schwab ME. Specific retrograde transport of nerve growth factor (NGF) from neocortex to nucleus basalis in the rat. *Brain Res* 1984; 300: 33–9.

(7) Dawbarn D, Allen SJ, Semenenko FM. Immunohistochemical localization of β-nerve growth factor receptors in the forebrain of the rat. *Brain Res* 1988; 440: 185–9.

(8) Gomez-Pinilla F, Cotman CW, Nieto-Sampedro M. NGF receptor immunoreactivity in rat brain: Topographic distribution and response to entorhinal ablation. *Neurosci Lett* 1987; 82: 260–6.

(9) Springer JE, Koh S, Tayrien MW, Loy R. Basal forebrain magnocellular neurons stain for nerve growth factor receptor: Correlation with cholinergic cell bodies and effects of axotomy. *J Neurosci Res* 1987; 17: 111–18.

(10) Dawbarn D, Allen SJ, Semenenko FM. Coexistence of choline acetyltransferase and β-nerve growth factor receptors in the forebrain of the rat. *Neurosci Lett* 1988; 94: 138–44.

(11) Allen SJ, Dawbarn D, Wilcock GK, Moss TH, Semenenko FM. The distribution of β-nerve growth factor receptors in the human basal forebrain. *J Comp Neurol* 1989; 289: 626–40.

(12) Hedreen JC, Struble RG, Whitehouse PJ, Price DL. Topography of the magnocellular basal forebrain system in human brain. *J Neuropathol Exp Neurol* 1984; 43: 1–21.

(13) Rossor MN, Svendsen C, Hunt SP, Mountjoy CQ, Roth M, Iversen LL. The substantia innominata in Alzheimer's disease: A histochemical and biochemical study of cholinergic marker enzymes. *Neurosci Lett* 1982; 28: 217–22.

(14) Saper CB, Chelimsky TC. A cytoarchitectonic and histochemical study of nucleus basalis and associated cell groups in the normal human brain. *Neuroscience* 1984; 13: 1023–37.

(15) German DC, Bruce G, Hersh LB. Immunohistochemical staining of cholinergic neurons in the human brain using the polyclonal antibody to human choline acetyltransferase. *Neurosci Lett* 1985; 61: 1–5.

(16) Mesulam MM, Geula C. Nucleus basalis (Ch4) and cortical cholinergic innervation in the human brain: observations based on the distribution of acetylcholinesterase and choline acetyltransferase. *J Comp Neurol* 1988; 275: 216–40.

(17) Nagai T, Pearson T, Heng F, McGeer EG, McGeer PL. Immunohistochemical staining of the human forebrain with monoclonal antibody to human choline acetyltransferase. *Brain Res* 1983; 265: 300–6.

(18) Pearson RCA, Sofroniew MV, Cuello AC et al. Persistence of cholinergic

D Dawbarn et al

neurons in the basal nucleus in a brain with senile dementia of the Alzheimer's type demonstrated by immunohistochemical staining for choline acetyltransferase. *Brain Res* 1983; 289: 375–9.

(19) Mobley WC, Rutkowski JL, Tennekoon GI, Gemski J, Buchanan K, Johnston MV. Nerve growth factor increases choline acetyltransferase activity in developing basal forebrain neurons. *Mol Brain Res* 1986; 1: 53–62.

(20) Mobley WC, Rutkowski JL, Tennekoon GI, Buchanan K, Johnston MV. Choline acetyltransferase activity in striatum of neonatal rats increased by nerve growth factor. *Science* 1986; 229: 284–7.

(21) Hefti F, Dravid A, Hartikka J. Chronic intraventricular injections of nerve growth factor elevate hippocampal choline acetyltransferase activity in adult rats with partial septohippocampal lesions. *Brain Res* 1984; 293: 305–11.

(22) Honnegar P, Lenoir D. Nerve growth factor (NGF) stimulation of cholinergic telencephalic neurons in aggregating cell cultures. *Dev Brain Res* 1982; 3: 229–38.

(23) Hefti H, Hartikka J, Eckenstein F, Gnahn H, Heumann R, Schwab M. Nerve growth factor (NGF) increases choline acetyltransferase but not survival or fiber growth of cultured septal cholinergic neurons. *Neuroscience* 1985; 14: 55–68.

(24) Martinez HJ, Dreyfus CF, Jonakeit M, Black IB. Nerve growth factor promotes cholinergic development in brain striatal cultures. *Proc Nat Acad Sci USA* 1985; 82: 7777–81.

(25) Gage FH, Armstrong DM, Williams LR, Varon S. Morphological response of axotomised septal neurons to nerve growth factor. *J Comp Neurol* 1988; 269: 147–55.

(26) Hagg T, Manthorpe M, Vahlsing HL, Varon S. Delayed treatment with nerve growth factor reverses the apparent loss of cholinergic neurons after acute brain damage. *Exp Neurol* 1988; 101: 303–12.

(27) Williams LR, Varon S, Peterson GM et al. Continuous infusion of nerve growth factor prevents basal forebrain neuronal death after fimbria-fornix transection. *Proc Nat Acad Sci USA* 1986; 83: 9231–5.

(28) Kromer LF. Nerve growth factor treatment after brain injury prevents neuronal death. *Science* 1987; 235: 214–16.

(29) Tuszyinski MH, UH-S, Amaral DG, Gage FH. Nerve growth factor infusion in the primate brain reduces lesion-induced cholinergic neuronal degeneration. *J Neurosci* 1990; 10: 3604–14.

(30) Koliatsos VE, Clatterbuck RE, Nauta HJ et al. Human nerve growth factor prevents degeneration of basal forebrain cholinergic neurons in primates. *Ann Neurol* 1991; 30: 831–40.

(31) Mandel RJ, Gage FH, Thal LJ. Spatial learning in rats: correlation with cortical choline acetyltransferase and improvement with NGF following NBM damage. *Exp Neurol* 1989; 104: 208–17.

(32) Fischer W, Wictorin A, Bjorklund A, Williams LR, Varon S, Gage FH. Amelioration of cholinergic neuronal atrophy and spatial memory impairment in aged rats by NGF. *Nature* 1987; 329: 65–7.

(33) Davies P. Neurotransmitter-related enzymes in senile dementia of the Alzheimer type. *Lancet* 1979; 171: 319–27.

(34) Allen SJ, Dawbarn D, MacGowan SH, Wilcock GK, Treanor JJS, Moss TH. A quantitative morphometric analysis of basal forebrain neurons expressing β-NGF receptors in normal and Alzheimer's disease brains. *Dementia* 1990; 1: 125–37.

(35) Hefti F, Mash DC. Localization of nerve growth factor receptors in the normal human brain and in Alzheimer's disease. *Neurobiol Aging* 1989; 10: 75–87.

(36) Mufson EJ, Bothwell M, Kordower JH. Loss of nerve growth factor receptor-containing neurons in Alzheimer's disease: a quantitative analysis across subregions of the basal forebrain. *Exp Neurol* 1989; 105: 221–32.

(37) Kordower JH, Gash DM, Bothwell M, Hersh LB, Mufson EJ. Nerve growth factor receptor and choline acetyltransferase remain colocalized in the nucleus basalis (Ch4) of Alzheimer's patients. *Neurobiol Aging* 1989; 10: 67–74.

(38) Perry EK, Perry RH, Gibson PH, Blessed G, Tomlinson BE. A cholinergic connection between normal aging and senile dementia in the human hippocampus. *Neurosci Lett* 1977; 6: 85–9.

(39) Goedert M, Fine A, Hunt SP, Ullrich A. Nerve growth factor mRNA in peripheral and central rat tissues and in the human central nervous system: lesion effects in the rat brain and levels in Alzheimer's disease. *Mol Brain Res* 1986; 1: 85–92.

(40) Wilcock GK, Esiri MM, Bowen DM, Smith CCT. The nucleus basalis in Alzheimer's disease: cell counts and cortical biochemistry. *Neuropathol Appl Neurobiol* 1983; 9: 175–9.

(41) Mesulam MM, Mufson EJ, Levey AI, Wainer BH. Cholinergic innervation of cortex by the basal forebrain: cytochemistry and cortical connections of the septal area, diagonal band nuclei, nucleus basalis (substantia innominata), and hypothalamus in the rhesus monkey. *J Comp Neurol* 1983; 214: 170–97.

(42) Goedert M, Fine A, Dawbarn D, Wilcock GK, Chao MV. Nerve growth factor receptor mRNA distribution in human brain: normal levels in basal forebrain in Alzheimer's disease. *Mol Brain Res* 1989; 5: 1–7.

(43) Treanor JJS, Dawbarn D, Allen SJ, MacGowan SH, Wilcock GK. Nerve growth factor receptor binding in normal and Alzheimer's disease basal forebrain. *Neurosci Lett* 1991; 121: 73–6.

(44) Mobley WC, Schenker A, Shooter EM. Characterization and isolation of proteolytically modified nerve growth factor. *Biochemistry* 1976; 25: 5543–52.

(45) Vale RD, Shooter EM. Assaying of nerve growth factor to cell surface receptors. *Meth Enzymol* 1985; 109: 21–39.

(46) Fabricant FN, De Larco JE, Todaro GJ. Nerve growth factor receptors on human melanoma cells in culture. *Proc Nat Acad Sci USA* 1977; 74: 565–9.

(47) Schecter AL, Bothwell MA. Nerve growth factor receptors on PC12 cells: evidence for two receptor classes with differing cytoskeletal associations. *Cell* 1981; 24: 867–74.

(48) Sutter A, Riopelle RJ, Harris-Warrick RM, Shooter EM. Nerve growth factor receptors. Characterization of two distinct classes of binding sites on chick embryo sensor ganglia cells. *J Biol Chem* 1979; 254: 5972–82.

(49) Riopelle RJ, Verge VMK, Richardson PM. Properties of receptors for nerve growth factor in mature rat nervous system. *Mol Brain Res* 1987; 3: 45–53.

D Dawbarn et al

(50) Larkfors L, Ebendal T, Whittmore SR, Persson H, Hoffer B, Olson L. Decreased level of nerve growth factor (NGF) and its messenger RNA in the aged rat brain. *Mol Brain Res* 1987; 3: 55–60.

(51) Korsching S, Thoenen H. Nerve growth factor in sympathetic ganglia and corresponding target organs of the rat: correlation with density of sympathetic innervation. *Proc Nat Acad Sci USA* 1985; 80: 3513–6.

(52) Hellweg R, Hock C, Hartung H-D. An improved rapid and highly sensitive enzyme immunoassay for nerve growth factor. In: *Technique – a journal of methods in cell and molecular biology* 1989; 1: 43–9.

(53) Allen SJ, MacGowan SH, Treanor JJS, Feeney R, Wilcock GK, Dawbarn D. Normal NGF content in Alzheimer's disease cerebral cortex and hippocampus. *Neurosci Lett* 1991; 131: 135–9.

(54) Barnett J, Baecker P, Routledge-Ward C et al. Human β-nerve growth factor obtained from a baculovirus expression system has potent in vitro and in vivo neurotrophic activity. *Exp Neurol* 1990; 110: 11–24.

(55) Scott SM, Selby M, Urdea M, Quiroga M, Bell GI, Rutter WJ. Isolation and nucleotide sequence of a cDNA clone encoding the precursor of mouse nerve growth factor. *Nature* 1983; 302: 538–40.

(56) Whittemore SR, Friedman PL, Larhammar D, Persson H, Gonzalez-Carvajal M, Holets VR. Rat beta-nerve growth factor sequence and site of synthesis in the adult hippocampus. *J Neurosci Res* 1988; 20: 403–10.

(57) Meier R, Becker-André M, Götz R, Heumann R, Shaw A, Thoenen H. Molecular cloning of bovine and chick nerve growth factor (NGF): delineation of conserved and unconserved domains and their relationship to the biological activity and antigenicity of NGF. *EMBO J* 1986; 5: 1489–93.

(58) Ullrich A, Gray A, Berman C, Dull TJ. Human β-nerve growth factor gene sequence highly homologous to that of mouse. *Nature* 1983; 303: 821–5.

(59) Leibrock J, Lottspeich F, Hohn A et al. Molecular cloning and expression of brain-derived neurotrophic factor. *Nature* 1989; 341: 149–52.

(60) Rosenthal A, Goeddel DV, Nguyen T et al. Primary structure and biological activity of human brain-derived neurotrophic factor. *Endocrinology* 1991; 129: 1289–94.

(61) Maisonpierre PC, LeBeau MM, Espinosa III R et al. Human and rat brain-derived neurotrophic factor and neurotrophin-3: gene structure, distributions and chromosomal localisations. *Genomics* 1991; 10: 558.

(62) Maisonpierre PC, Belluscio L, Squinto S et al. Neurotrophin-3: a neurotrophic factor related to NGF and BDNF. *Science* 1990; 247: 1446–51.

(63) Rosenthal A, Goeddel DV, Nguyen T et al. Primary structure and biological activity of a novel human neurotrophic factor. *Neuron* 1990; 4: 767–73.

(64) Ernfors P, Ibanez CF, Ebendal T, Olsen L, Persson H. Molecular cloning and neurotrophic activities of a protein with structural similarities to nerve growth factor: developmental and topographical expression in the brain. *Proc Nat Acad Sci USA* 1990; 87: 5454–8.

(65) Kaisho Y, Yoshimora K, Nakahama K. Cloning and expression of a cDNA encoding a novel human neurotrophic factor. *FEBS Lett* 1990; 266: 187–91.

(66) Hallbook F, Ibanez CF, Persson H. Evolutionary studies of the nerve growth

factor family reveal a novel member abundantly expressed in *Xenopus* ovary. *Neuron* 1991; 6: 845–58.

(67) Berkmeir LR, Winslow JW, Kaplan DR, Nikolics K, Goeddel DV, Rosenthal R. Neurotrophin-5 – a novel neurotrophic factor that activates trk and trkB. *Neuron* 1991; 7: 857–66.

(68) Ip N, Ibanez CF, Nye SH et al. Mammalian neurotrophin-4: structure, chromosomal localisation, tissue distribution and receptor specificity. *Proc Nat Acad Sci USA* 1992; 89: 3060–4.

(69) McDonald NQ, Lapatto R, Murray-Rust J, Gunning J, Wlodawer A, Blundell TL. New protein fold revealed by a 2.3-Å resolution crystal structure of nerve growth factor.

(70) Uri Saragovi H, Greene MI, Chrusciel RA, Kahn M. Loops and secondary structure mimetics: development and applications and basic science and rational drug design. *Bio/technol* 1992; 10: 773–8.

(71) Greene LA, Tischler AS. Establishment of a noradrenergic clonal line of rat adrenal pheochromocytoma cells which respond to nerve growth factor. *Proc Nat Acad Sci USA* 1976; 73: 2424–8.

(72) Bernd P, Greene LA. Association of ^{125}I-nerve growth factor with PC12 pheochromocytoma cells. Evidence for internalization via high affinity receptors only and for long-term regulation by nerve growth factor of both high and low affinity receptors. *J Biol Chem* 1984; 259: 15509–16.

(73) Massague J, Guilette BJ, Czech MP, Morgan CJ, Bradshaw RA. Identification of a nerve growth factor receptor protein in sympathetic ganglia membranes by affinity labelling. *J Biol Chem* 1981; 256: 9419–24.

(74) Meakin SO, Shooter EM. Molecular investigations on the high affinity nerve growth factor receptor. *Neuron* 1991; 6: 153–63.

(75) Martin-Zanca D, Hughes SH, Barbacid M. A human oncogene formed by the fusion of truncated tropomysin and protein tyrosine kinase sequences. *Nature* 1986; 319: 743–8.

(76) Martin-Zanca D, Oskam R, Mitra G, Copeland T, Barbacid M. Molecular and biochemical characterization of the human trk proto-oncogene. *Mol Cell Biol* 1989; 9: 24–33.

(77) Klein R, Parada LF, Coulier F, Barbacid M. trkB, a novel tyrosine kinase receptor expressed during mouse neural development. *EMBO J* 1989; 8: 3701–9.

(78) Klein R, Conway D, Parada LF, Barbacid M. The trkB tyrosine protein kinase gene codes for a second neurogenic receptor that lacks the catalytic kinase domain. *Cell* 1990; 61: 647–56.

(79) Middlemas DS, Lindberg RA, Hunter T. trkB, a neural receptor protein-tyrosine kinase: evidence for a full-length and two truncated receptors. *Mol Cell Biol* 1991; 11: 143–53.

(80) Lamballe F, Klein R, Barbacid M. trkC, a new member of the trk family of tyrosine protein kinases, is a receptor for neurotrophin-3. *Cell* 1991; 66: 967–79.

(81) Kaplan DR, Martin-Zanca D, Parada LF. Tyrosine phosphorylation and tyrosine kinase activity of the trk proto-oncogene induced by NGF. *Nature* 1991; 350: 158–60.

(82) Klein R, Jing S, Nanduri V, O'Rourke E, Barbacid M. The trk proto-oncogene encodes the receptor for nerve growth factor. *Cell* 1991; 65: 189–97.

(83) Kaplan DR, Hempstead BL, Martin-Zanca D, Chao MV, Parada LF. The trk proto-oncogene product: a signal transducing receptor for nerve growth factor. *Science* 1991; 252: 554–8.

(84) Hempstead BL, Martin-Zanca D, Kaplan DR, Parada LF, Chao MV. High affinity NGF binding requires co-expression of the trk proto-oncogene and the low affinity NGF receptor. *Nature* 1991; 350: 678–83.

(85) Squinto SP, Stitt TN, Aldrich TH et al. trkB encodes a functional receptor for brain-derived neurotrophic receptor and neurotrophin-3 but not nerve growth factor. *Cell* 1991; 65: 885–93.

(86) Soppet D, Escandon E, Maragos J et al. The neurotrophic factors brain-derived neurotrophic factor and neurotrophin-3 are ligands for the trkB tyrosine kinase receptor. *Cell* 1991; 65: 895–903.

(87) Glass DJ, Nye SH, Hantzopoulos P et al. trkB mediates BDNF/NT-3 dependent survival and proliferation in fibroblasts lacking the low affinity NGF receptor. *Cell* 1991; 66: 405–13.

(88) Klein R, Lamballe F, Bryant S, Barbacid M. The trikB tyrosine protein kinase is a receptor for neurotrophin-4. *Neuron* 1992; 8: 947–56.

(89) Martin-Zanca D, Barbacid M, Parada LF. Expression of the *trk* proto-oncogene is restricted to the sensory cranial and spinal ganglia of neural crest origin in mouse development. *Genes Dev* 1990; 4: 683–94.

(90) Nebrada AR, Martin-Zanca D, Kaplan DR, Parada LF, Santos E. Induction by NGF of meiotic maturation of xenopus oocytes expressing the trk proto-oncogene product. *Science* 1991; 252: 558–62.

(91) Cordon-Cardo C, Tapley T, Jing S et al. The trk tyrosine protein kinase mediates the mitogenic properties of nerve growth factor and neurotrophin-3. *Cell* 1991; 66: 173–83.

(92) Ibanez CF, Ebendal T, Barbany G, Murray-Rust J, Blundell TL, Persson H. Disruption of the low affinity binding site in NGF allows neuronal survival and differentiation by binding to the trk gene product. *Cell* 1992; 69: 329–41.

(93) Pleasure SJ, Reddy UR, Venkatakrisnan G et al. Introduction of nerve growth factor (NGF) receptor into a medulloblastoma cell line results in expression of high- and low-affinity NGF receptors but not NGF-mediated differentiation. *Proc Nat Acad Sci USA* 1990; 87: 8496–500.

(94) Hempstead BL, Schliefer LS, Chao MV. Expression of functional nerve growth factor receptors after gene transfer. *Science* 1989; 243: 373–5.

(95) Berg MM, Sternberg DW, Hempstead BL, Chao MV. The low affinity p75 nerve growth factor (NGF) receptor mediates NGF-induced tyrosine phosphorylation. *Proc Nat Acad Sci USA* 1991; 88: 7106–10.

(96) Rodriguez-Tebar A, Dechant G, Barde Y-A. Binding of brain-derived neurotrophic factor to the nerve growth factor receptor. *Neuron* 1990; 4: 487–92.

(97) Rodriguez-Tebar A, Dechant G, Gotz R, Barde Y-A. Binding of neurotrophin-3 to its neuronal receptors and interactions with nerve growth factor and brain-derived neurotrophic factor. *EMBO J* 1992; 11: 917–22.

(98) Kuo-Fen L, Li En, Huber J et al. Targeted mutation of the gene encoding the

low affinity NGF receptor p75 leads to deficits in the peripheral sensory nervous system. *Cell* 1992; 69: 737–49.

(99) Wright EM, Vogel KS, Davies AM. Neurotrophic factors promote the maturation of developing sensory neurons before they become dependent on these factors for survival. *Neuron* 1992; 9: 139–50.

(100) Alderson RF, Alterman AL, Barde Y-A, Lindsey RM. Brain-derived neurotrophic factor increases survival and differentiated functions of rat septal cholinergic neurons in culture. *Neuron* 1990; 5: 297–306.

(101) Phillips HS, Hains JM, Armanini M, Laramee GR, Johnson SA, Winslow JW. BDNF mRNA is decreased in the hippocampus of individuals with Alzheimer's disease. *Neuron* 1991; 7: 695–702.

(102) Olson L, Nordberg A, von Holst H et al. Nerve growth factor affects ^{11}C-nicotine binding, blood flow, EEG, and verbal episodic memory in Alzheimer patient. *J Neur Transmiss* 1992; 4: 79–95.

(103) Hyman C, Hofer M, Barde Y-A et al. BDNF is a neurotrophic factor for dopaminergic neurons of the substantia nigra. *Nature* 1991; 350: 230–2.

(104) Knusel B, Winslow JW, Rosenthal A et al. Promotion of central cholinergic and dopaminergic neuron differentiation by brain-derived neurotrophic factor but not neurotrophin-3. *Proc Nat Acad Sci USA* 1991; 88: 961–5.

The biology of mental handicap

A J HOLLAND

Introduction

Normal human development from conception to adult life follows a path which is, by and large, predictable. During fetal life this is characterized by the systematic differentiation of separate organ systems and parts of the body, leading to the development of a viable fetus at the time of birth. In children, this developmental process continues through the growth and physical development of the child, and can be observed in the reaching of particular developmental milestones such as smiling, sitting, standing, walking and the complex process of language development. The passing of these milestones is associated with the development of more advanced skills such as being able to dress, and the acquisition of other abilities such as literacy and numeracy skills. During childhood, not only do the basic skills necessary for a normal life develop but the more subtle and complex attributes of human beings also become apparent. This is exemplified by the Piagetian stages of development. For example, the development of the ability to engage in symbolic play and to understand and communicate complex ideas and feelings through an increasingly sophisticated language.

Within a given population, there will always be variation in the precise timing of these developmental milestones because of both the inherent differences between individuals and the differences in individual environments. The process of development is an interactive one, the relative contributions of biologically and environmentally determined factors changing over time[1]. For instance, babies and young children require stimulation. Without this, acquisition of new skills is delayed and, in cases of abuse and neglect, particular patterns of impaired language development are observed[2]. What is unclear is whether such stimulation has a direct impact on neural development and thus on skills development or whether stimulation simply enables a skill to become apparent which is in fact, in neural terms, already feasible. The possible importance of early childhood stimulation has resulted in program-

All correspondence to: Dr A J Holland, Academic Department of Psychiatry, Addenbrooke's Hospital, Hills Road, Cambridge CB2 2QQ, UK

Cambridge Medical Reviews: Neurobiology and Psychiatry Volume 2
© Cambridge University Press

mes designed to give children with disabilities or who come from socially deprived backgrounds a 'head start'. Interestingly, studies of such programmes, particularly in children with biologically determined developmental disorders, are inconclusive and add further fuel to the nature/nurture debate[3].

The growth and development of the brain, and of the individual a a whole, can be a hazardous process, and problems in brain development at any stage may predispose an individual to eventual abnormal mental and intellectual development. Although this process of development is fundamentally dependent on normal brain development, there are factors such as later educational and social influences and the process of experience which may smooth the negative effects of abnormal brain development on subsequent intellectual and social abilities and mental state[4]. It is therefore an enormously difficult task when trying to disentangle the various influences giving rise to the presence of, or lack of, particular social and living skills, complex cognitive abilities and/or the capacity to understand and anticipate the thoughts and feelings of others, which characterize human beings.

This chapter is concerned with understanding the factors of biological origin which give rise to the presence of a 'handicap' which has affected a person's ability to learn, to acquire living and social skills and to reason and communicate through language. The starting point is first to discuss what is meant by the term 'mental handicap', secondly to assess what is known about the development of the human central nervous system (CNS) following conception and finally to discuss some of the known genetic, chromosomal and environmental influences which may impede or impair normal brain development and result in mental handicap.

This chapter tries to provide a framework within which it is possible to consider the impact of biologically determined factors on the ultimate intellectual and emotional development of an individual. Given that people who are mentally handicapped have an increased risk of developing additional behavioural and psychiatric disorders[5-8], there is also the further questions of how these factors might have contributed to the disordered behaviour, or to the presence of a mental illness which has brought this person in contact with specialist mental health services.

What is mental handicap?

The term 'mental handicap' is used when the process of childhood development is delayed or deviant so that some or all of the milestones are delayed as well as the acquisition of skills, and the development of more complex intellectual abilities. This definition is purposely broad and therefore cannot adequately describe the heterogeneity of this group of people. Some have a severe mental handicap and have acquired very few skills and very limited language development. For this group of 0.3% to 0.4% of the general population, lifelong support will be necessary[9]. For others the newer term of 'learn-

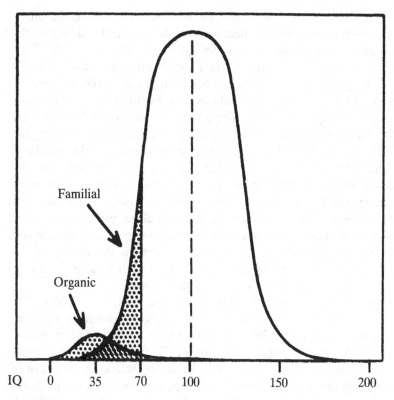

Fig. 1. Diagram illustrating the near normal distribution of IQ scores within an unselected population. Approximately 2% of the population have scores more than two standard deviations below the mean (IQ <70). This group are at risk for mental handicap. The skew to the left is due to the occurrence of specific disorders which adversely affect brain development.

ing disability' is more appropriate as early development may not be markedly different from an accepted normal range, the disability becoming apparent only at school where assessment of their intellectual ability is shown to fall within the low few per cent of the population. Furthermore, in addition to considerable variation in intellectual ability, individuals within this group vary in the precise nature of their developmental disability and the presence or not of additional disabilities. For example, specific impairments of social and language development characteristic of autism may be present[10], sensory impairments are more common[11] and with increasing levels of impairment the rates of epilepsy increase to approximately 50%[12].

Fig. 1 illustrates the near normal distribution of IQ scores in an unselected population. The observed skew to the left is due to the occurrence of specific disorders, for example Down's syndrome, which are almost invariably associated with intellectual impairment and the presence of a learning disability. These disorders have a marked effect on brain development and thus on the potential intellectual development of the individual. This 2% to 3% of the population whose IQ are two standard deviations below the mean IQ represent the group 'at risk' for mental handicap. Their intellectual abilities are limited but other factors may influence the extent of any resultant disability and handicap (see below). The level of handicap will be dependent upon the outcome of a number of different interactive factors including the biologically determined effects on brain development, early childhood opportunities for education and help in the acquisition of skills and the individual's present circumstances. For some, the abnormality of brain development which is due, for example, to the presence of a chromosomal abnormality, sets clear limitations to intellectual development and the ultimate level of skills acquisition. In these circumstances lifelong care and support will be required but within these limitations the quality of the environment, and an understanding of individual need leading to specific intervention can maximize an individual's quality of life.

Different systems of classification have emphasized different aspects. For example, in the USA the emphasis is on the 'adaptive behaviour' of a person, and his or her ability to develop new living and social skills. Other systems continue to rely on standardized measures of IQ, for example, the international classification of diseases, ICD 9[13]. An understanding of the extent of any biologically or environmentally determined influence on an individual's handicap requires an appropriate conceptual framework. The World Health Organization[14] classification system of impairments, disabilities and handicaps is a hierarchic framework which can provide the basis for a more sophisticated analysis of the extent to which different factors contribute to the ultimate level of handicap. Handicap is not simply seen as a consequence of a particular disease process but as an interaction between such a process and the level of intervention, and the extent to which the environment can be changed to minimize the handicap. In this system of classification, it is the 'impairment' which is considered to be the 'exteriorization' of a pathological state and 'disability' is the loss of ability consequent upon the impairment[15]. Within this framework of classification, mental handicap can be seen to be due to a disorder of development in which the fundamental impairment is primarily that of cognition and intellectual ability. In the case of disorders which have a major effect on brain development, there are invariably other severe impairments affecting acquisition of skills. It is within the understanding of the factors which influence the level and type of 'impairments' where the neurobiologists and geneticists have the greatest contribution to make.

There are many different reasons for a person being mentally handicapped. In some cases, the abnormality of brain development is understood but, in others, it is far from clear and the questions remain as to whether each disorder (genetic, chromosomal or environmental in origin) has a unique effect or whether there may be a final common pathway by which a number of different disorders have their effect on the developing CNS. There has also been a very extensive debate as to whether these disorders result in 'delayed' or 'deviant' development. This 'developmental' perspective has increasingly informed thinking in the field of 'mental retardation'[16]. It is argued that normal development is an active process in which change occurs, resulting in specific endpoints and changing mental schemas or concepts due to both qualitative and quantitative neuropsychological changes. In this context distinctions have been drawn between mental handicap of 'organic' and 'familial' origins. In the case of the former, CNS development may be 'deviant', and in the latter, 'delayed'. Others have argued that there may be common principles which underlie the developmental process, regardless of whether there is an apparent disorder of development or not. The arguments for, and against, the different perspectives are complex, but comparisons between disorders such as autism[17], or the study of the cognitive development of people with Down's syndrome[18] or those with Fragile-X syndrome[19,20], clearly indicate that 'mental handicap' is not a unitary phenomenon which can be conveniently pigeonholed into one box. From the perspective of research, as well as from the point of view of intervention, there are clear differences in the 'developmental profile' and therefore, presumably, the pattern of brain development, between people with different developmental disorders, even if the level of intellectual impairment is similar. The neural basis for such differences are inevitably going to be very complex and how such differences might be identified at the level of neuronal structure and function may be beyond our present capabilities. However, the study of CNS development has identified some important mechanisms, which if defective can result in CNS abnormalities, ranging from the obvious to the very subtle. These in turn, might predispose to the differences referred to above.

Human central nervous system development

As with any other organ in the human body the central nervous system develops from undifferentiated cells which have become differentiate initially into the ectoderm and later still into increasingly specialized cells. The formation of the neural plate leads to the development of the neural folds which become increasingly pronounced and eventually form the neural tube. During this process of neurulation, mesodermal structures are also beginning to form, such as the notochord which eventually becomes the spinal column. As the neural tube closes, the neural crest cells begin to give rise to the peripheral nervous system and nonneural tissue. There is little cell division at this early stage of neurulation but changes in cell shape and cell adhesion may be of particular importance[21]. The brain itself is formed as a result of the development of fore-, mid- and hindbrain vesicles at the rostral end of the neural tube, developing into the cerebral hemispheres, midbrain and lower brain stem respectively. These changes are due primarily to the rapid proliferation of cells differentially at the rostral end of the neural tube. It has been estimated that at this stage 250 000 neurones per minute are being added, resulting in the eventual estimated 100 billion neurones of the human brain. With this rapid proliferation of cells, particularly of the forebrain, a process of complex folding takes place leading to the final structure of the brain (see Fig. 2)[22].

The development of the nervous system does not take place in isolation but within the context of the developing organism as a whole and therefore is both influenced by and influences developing sensory and motor systems. In addition, there is a changing metabolic and hormonal environment. It is difficult to disentangle, on the one hand, the direct effect of gene expression itself on this process to, on the other, the influence of the intra- and extracellular environment then created, on subsequent gene expression and, in turn, on the growth and differentiation of the neurones and glial cells which make up the functioning nervous system. At least three categories of influence at this early stage are thought to be important. These include the instructions contained within the nucleus, ie genes and other DNA, the influence of cytoplasmic structures and proteins which effect gene expression, and instructions arising from other developing cells and the extracellular environment (for example, cell adhesion molecules, trophic factors and neuronal activity itself). The interaction between these broad categories of influence also change over time with, for example, the switching on and off of gene expression and with the increasing sophistication of the neuronal environment.

This process of differentiation takes place during the first 20 weeks of fetal life. At an early stage, before cell migration begins, glial and neuronal cells, although having a common origin, can be shown to have begun differentiation by the presence of a specific glial protein in some but not other cells[23]. The neurones which grow at this time cannot be replaced but are the basis for all future brain function. They may have a lifespan of 70 or more years. However, during their lifetime they have to change in subtle ways in order to reflect the process of learning, and of mental activity. Animal research has identified a number of principles which may be important in the process whereby neurones travel considerable distances but ultimately appear to make the connections which allow a functioning neural network to become established. Study of the development of the nervous system in the roundworm Caenorhabditis elegans has demonstrated that there appears to be some element of preprogramming in that the growth and migration of some neurones does not appear to be affected by the ablation of neighbouring cells[24]. In other cases, the ablation of one neurone results in the recruitment of another cell of equivalent lineage to take its place or in the proliferation of neighbouring cells[25,26]. In more advanced animals over 50 types of neurones (pyramidal,

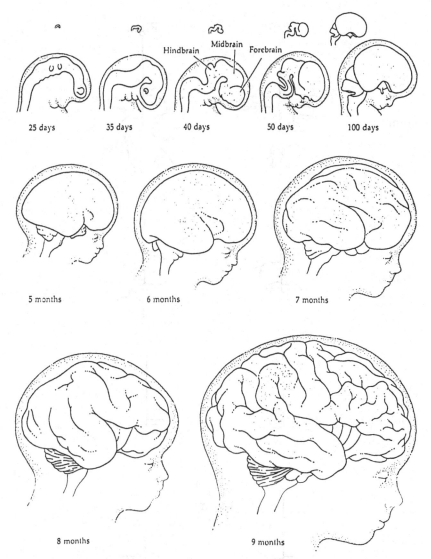

Fig. 2. Diagram illustrating the chronological development of the human brain. (Taken from Purves & Lichtman, 1985[22].) The top row of diagrams are not to scale.

stellate, purkinje, etc) have been described, all sharing some similar features but being characterized according to the varying numbers of cell processes and the extent of their projections, for example, whether they project within or between cerebral nuclei. There appears to be some intrinsic basis for this specialization as in tissue culture neurones from particular nuclei have an approximately similar shape[27]. In addition, neurons from genetically identical animals have been shown to be similar but not identical[28] (see Fig. 3).

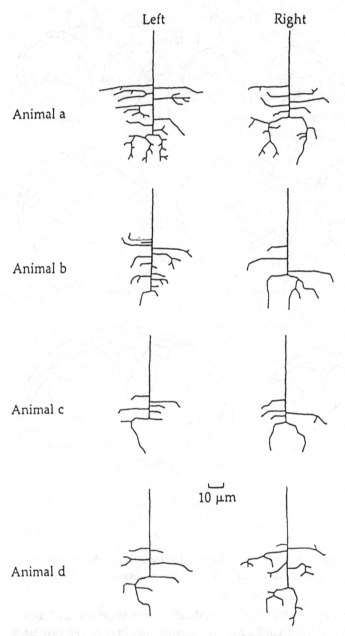

Fig. 3. Dendritic branching patterns of homologous neurones on the left and right side of the optic ganglion neuropil in four water fleas. All four animals were genetically identical. There is variability in the pattern of the neurones both between genetically identical animals and also between the left and right side of the same animals indicating that neuronal branching is not completely under genetic control. (Taken from Purves & Lichtman, 1985 [22].)

Neurones have to migrate along radial glial fibres ending considerable distances from their place of origin. They therefore have to make contact with glial cells and their subsequent viability and successful migration is dependent upon the properties of 'cell adhesion' molecules[29]. Gadisseux et al.[30] studied the migration of neurones in fetal mice in relationship to the network of radial glial fibres. They described changes in the glial structure through the cortical wall and a relative selective relationship between specific migratory neurones and radial glial fibres. There is also a pattern to this migration so that in the cortex the outer and inner cortical layers are formed from the first cells to migrate and the central layers from the later migratory cells. Thus particular cortical abnormalities found associated with specific syndromes can be classified according to whether they are due to a failure of early or late migration or are postmigratory in origin.

Broad categories of abnormalities can be identified. Microcephaly, which has many possible causes such as maternal phenylketonuria[31] or autosomal and sex linked disorders, may be due to a reduction in the total number of neurones or to a failure of migration of neurones[32]. Other focal disorders of brain development may be due to abnormalities of neuronal migration giving rise to heterotopias and focal cortical dysplasias. Thus it becomes possible to see how such cerebral abnormalities, regardless of their fundamental cause, may result in superficially similar to markedly different clinical pictures according to whether the resultant underlying cerebral abnormality is similar or different.

The migration of neurones over considerable distances is followed by the development of extensive connections with neighbouring cells through dendrite formation and the eventual formation of synaptic vesicles. It appears that different classes of neurones have different periods of sensitivity to nerve growth factor (NGF). For example, sympathetic nerve cells can fail to branch and develop if NGF is inactivated through the use of an antisera, or can grow excessively if NGF is given in excess[33]. This was not found to be the case with dorsal root ganglion cells although they grow if treated with NGF in vitro[34]. It has therefore been proposed that NGF is important for the further growth of neurones following migration but the effect may be limited to a particular period in the cells' development. A rare autosomal recessive disorder, familial dysautonomia, is thought to be due to NGF dysfunction[35] and other disorders, including some related to abnormal intellectual development, could be similarly related to a failure of appropriate neuronal connections due to abnormalities in the NGF system[36].

In the second half of pregnancy, there is a considerable growth of the brain associated with other maturational changes. Brain weight increases from 10 g at 20 weeks gestation to 350 g at term and 950 g at the end of the first year postnatally. In addition, it has been shown that there is a change in the previously established dendritic connections with the loss of axons and a rationalization of the neural networks[37]. This is possibly related to activity-dependent competition between axonal inputs for common postsynaptic neurons[38]. This has been referred to as the 'subtractive' phase of brain development in contrast to the previous 'additive' phase. The latter results in the major structures and connections of the CNS being established, whereas the former allows for the correction of redundant or incorrect connections and for the refining of connections. Many of these conclusions have been arrived at from the study of the development of the visual system in primates and other mammals. This neural system has provided the model for what might be presumed to be the basis of the maturational process which occurs following neuronal migration as well as for investigating the influence of external sensory experience on neural development[39]. Axons from retinal ganglion cells of both eyes project to the lateral geniculate nuclei (LGN) on both sides of the brain and axons from the LGN project from there to layer four of the primary visual cortex. These projections both at the LGN and at the cortex at first show no specific pattern relating to the eye of origin. However, eye specific layers in both the LGN and the primary visual cortex begin to emerge as a process of remodelling takes place[40]. In higher mammals, the remodelling of the LGN input occurs prenatally but in the cortex, postnatally[41]. In humans, neurones in the primary visual cortex are primarily binocularly driven, apart from in layer four of the cortex which remain primarily monocular. However, it is clear that the function of neurones in the primary visual cortex is dependent upon an input from both eyes. If the eyelid to one eye is closed postnatally then, when it is reopened, that eye no longer drives neurones in the primary visual cortex[42]. However, neurones in the LGN and retina remain responsive[43]. Anatomical changes can also be observed in the LGN indicating that transient deprivation of a sensory input has a profound effect on structure and function at least during a 'critical period'[39]. Further studies involving the use of drugs which block neuronal transmission have demonstrated the importance of sensory input in the development and refining of the visual system[44]. However, such input is not always essential as spontaneous firing of neurones in the visual system has been observed even when animals are raised in the dark. Such neuronal activity results in changes in the LGN and primary visual cortex[45]. Furthermore, the response of the developing visual pathways to sensory input is not just due to presynaptic effects but can be enhanced by changes in postsynaptic activity[46]. Other neural systems have also been shown to exhibit the same effects in that their normal development is dependent upon patterns of neuronal input[47].

The process of moderation of the original axonal connections results in cell death and modification of dendritic connections[37]. This is thought to continue long after birth and synaptic density may be at its greatest in the first year of life[48] decreasing through childhood. It is therefore possible that increasingly complex sensory inputs influence this process. The time in fetal or postfetal life that the modification occurs varies between different areas of the brain, the visual system being before the prefrontal cortex[49,50]. This in turn may mirror cognitive developments.

The above observations on the development of the visual system in particular illustrate two important points. First, these studies support the idea that neuronal connections are refined on the basis of 'use-dependent synaptic competition'. Secondly, they and other studies suggest that there is plasticity in the development of the CNS but only for particular periods of time. The research which was able to demonstrate these effects has used severe methods to restrict visual input, eg sewing up the eyelids and the relevance to understanding the cognitive deficits of people with developmental disorder is open to question. For example, severe adversity in childhood appears to have relatively few long-term consequences[51] and in the absence of additional biological factors such deprivation is not a major contribution to the etiology of mental handicap. However, studies of auditory discrimination suggest that a critical period within which children learn to distinguish phonemes unique to a specific language does exist[52,53]. Furthermore, sensory impairments are not infrequently associated with specific mental handicapping syndromes and therefore in addition to any developmental disorder of the brain, impaired sensory input may also affect development. It is also possible that impairment in function of one particular neuronal network might in turn result in a failure of normal development of another and so on. Thus deficits compound. Whether there is a 'critical period' for the development of more complex abilities therefore is open to question but study of the visual system does indicate that there are 'critical' periods in the development of some of the more advanced functions of the visual system. These differ in their timing from earlier levels of development of visual perception, indicating that a similar process of interactive development occurs even with the acquisition of more complex visual abilities[54].

As mentioned earlier in this chapter, CNS development is taking place in a continually changing environment. In utero, this is both maternally and fetally determined and the passage of viruses, excessive maternal alcohol consumption or, for example, excessive amounts of phenylalanine as occurs in maternal phenylketonuria, can result in severely impaired CNS development and mental handicap (see below). In addition, the fetal environment is changing, and the male and female sex hormones and other hormones may influence brain development, and could account for the excess of some disabilities in males compared to females. Although it is clear from the early work of Penrose[55], and with the continuing reporting of X-linked disorders that this accounts for some of the excess, it is unlikely to explain the higher rates of, for example, autism in boys, or of other specific developmental disabilities. Influences, including those of the sex hormones, which affect cerebral lateralization have been reviewed by Geschwind and Galaburda[56].

The brain is the basis for all mental activity. If its development is impaired or abnormal, there then exists the potential for abnormalities of normal cognitive and mental abilities and emotional experience. This brief examination of the process of CNS development from conception to adult life illustrates how there exists at many different points the possibility of error. Genes and/or their controlling DNA sequences may be absent or have a point mutation. There may be failure of the normal differentiation and folding of the neural tube. Neuronal migration may be faulty. Neuronal cell division may be abnormal or delayed thus affecting brain growth. There may be a failure of normal rationalization of neurone numbers and dendritic structure. Impaired sensory input may, in turn, affect normal neuronal development. In many of the rarer single gene disorders, the mechanism whereby the brain is affected is directly related to the absence of a particular enzyme and therefore the abnormal storage of metabolites in brain cells, eg the lysosomal storage diseases. In other disorders, the actual mechanism whereby brain function becomes impaired is far from clear, although abnormalities of some of the above processes may be the final common pathway whereby particular abnormalities affect brain development and thus mental ability. Finally, if the development of different parts of the CNS are dependent upon patterns of neuronal activity, then a fault in one system may affect the development of another.

Biological causes of abnormal brain development and mental handicap

People who since childhood can be shown to fall in the low 2% to 3% of the population in terms of intellectual ability and level of functioning, can be said to have an intellectual impairment. They will invariably have a learning disability and are likely to be disadvantaged. The level of disability and subsequent handicap may be modified by maximizing an individual's ability through appropriate education, family support, and through changes in the environment that help to counteract the impact of limited literacy and numeracy skills, sensory impairments or physical disabilities. This group of people may well have been born with, or have acquired, a disorder which has impaired brain development. The detection of these disorders is important as knowing the cause may help parents accept their handicapped child, enable informed genetic counselling and/or specific treatments and may alert those concerned to the likely development of additional health problems in later life. Earlier methods of classification drew a distinction between relatively rare and 'syndrome' causes and familial factors. Lewis[57] argued that there was a distinction between those who had mild degrees of impairment for 'subcultural' reasons and those with undoubted organic disorders. In the former group, a combination of polygenic and environmentally determined factors contributed to the level of handicap and thus the intervention proposed by

Lewis was primarily educational and social in content. A similar distinction was made by Tredgold[58] who referred to primary and secondary causes. It is clear that those with mild intellectual impairment are unlikely to have a pathological syndrome. In general there is a familial correlation in IQ, unlike in severe mental handicap, indicating that mild intellectual impairment is polygenically determined[59]. Epidemiological studies such as the one carried out in Aberdeen supports this view. Birch et al.[60] reported that people with more severe disabilities had evidence of abnormal brain development on the basis of CNS examination. This group with evidence of CNS abnormalities and severe impairments were found across all social backgrounds. Whereas those with lesser degrees of impairment (divided according to IQ) were found to be in families in social classes iv and v. However, with increasingly sophisticated technologies (biochemical, cytogenetic and molecular genetic) combined with more sophisticated psychological assessment techniques, it has become clear that this division between organic and subcultural, and, in turn, between severe and mild degrees of impairment, respectively, is less distinct than originally anticipated. Those with mild impairments may have an identifiable disorder, eg female fragile-X carriers, and those with identifiable organic disorders, such as Down's syndrome, may only have a mild level of impairment.

It is not possible to cover in detail all the known causes of developmental intellectual impairments and mental handicap and chapters in general textbooks provide detailed information[61]. However, it is important to identify broad groups of disorders and to see how some of these may interfere with brain development. The three broad categories are the rare single gene disorders, numerical and structural abnormalities of sex chromosomes and the autosomes, and disorders due to environmental problems in utero or after birth including the teratogenic effects of viruses or maternal alcohol abuse, cerebral anoxia prior to or during birth or severe infections or injury during childhood. In addition, there are syndromes whose etiology is unknown and in some studies up to a third of individuals diagnosed as mentally handicapped had no established cause[62].

Single gene disorders
Of the 90 000 genes which are expressed in human beings, over half are thought to be expressed within the brain. Individual genes will be expressed in different cells, in different parts of the nervous system (for example, in specific CNS nuclei as well as different cell types) and at different times in the developmental process. In addition to genes which are expressed in the brain, other disorder may affect brain development and function, for example, lysosomal storage disorders. Within this group alone, 30 different variants have been described, many affecting the brain[63]. There is considerable genetic heterogeneity with single mutations of base pairs or deletions of whole

157

A J Holland

genes, parts of genes or controlling sequences reported, all of which may lead to a similar clinical manifestation[64]. In some of these disorders, it is clear that the pathological process is active in utero and even if the biochemical abnormality is understood, treatment would still prove very difficult.

Of probable single gene disorders associated with abnormal intellectual development 503 have been reported[65]. Of these 69 have been mapped to the autosomes and 73 to the X-chromosome. The remaining are unlocated. These disorders are invariably associated with other physical abnormalities and metabolic disturbances. It has been estimated that these may account for as little as 4% of the causes of developmental disorders[62]. Their identification is important so that genetic counselling and, in some cases, specific treatments can be offered to those affected. Phenylketonuria is the best example of such a disorder. Folling in 1934 identified the excessive levels of phenylalanine and concluded that this was a recessive disorder caused by the absence of an enzyme necessary for phenylalanine metabolism[64]. Cowie[66] described the full phenotype. Later the benefits of dietary restriction of phenylalanine were confirmed[67]. However, it is clear that even children who were identified shortly after birth and placed on an appropriate diet continue to have neuropsychological deficits particularly of visuospatial and visuomotor tasks[68]. These specific impairments may have a neurochemical basis and it has been argued that continuing phenylalanine restriction and/or tyrosine supplements may result in improvements[69].

Stern[64] points out that there have been considerable achievements in the understanding of the rare inborn errors of metabolism such as disorders of the Krebs cycle, glygogen storage diseases and a new class of disorders in which the metabolic deficit is within cell bodies called 'peroxisomes'[70]. However, although in theory treatment is sometimes possible with these disorders, the quality of life may be very poor and minor infections can be life threatening.

Chromosomal abnormalities
Since the first description of human chromosomes[71] it has been recognized that chromosomal abnormalities are an important cause of developmental disorders and mental handicap. Chromosomes can be visualized in the prophase or metaphase of the cell cycle. Many chromosomal abnormalities such as loss of autosomes or the inheritance of extra autosomes results in a nonviable fetus, or in such severe congenital anomalies, that life span is shortened. Approximately 50% of miscarriages and 1% of live born fetuses have been reported to have a chromosome abnormality[72]. Loss of or increase in sex chromosomes (XO, XYY, XXY, XXYY), trisomy 21, deletions and other structural rearrangement of chromosomes such as translocations are the most common chromosomal abnormalities in live born children, and are invariably associated with mild to more severe forms of learning disability. With improvements in cytogenetic techniques, and now with application of molec-

158

ular genetic methodologies, increasing numbers of deletions and other chromosomal rearrangements are being detected, such as the recently described thalassemmia/mental retardation syndromes[73]. Lamb et al.[74] have argued that such submicroscopic chromosomal abnormalities, particularly at the telomeres of chromosomes, may be an important but unrecognized cause of genetic disease. Fluorescent in situ hybridization (FISH) is a new technique which may help identify these chromosomal abnormalities which are thought to occur particularly at the telomeres of chromosomes because of the presence of repeat base pair sequences, thus giving rise to the possibility of mispairing[75,76].

The mechanisms whereby chromosomal abnormalities give rise to disorders of development are unclear. In cases of chromosomal rearrangements or small deletions, the effect may be due to the loss or disruption of expression of a single gene. Where there is multiple pathology, the phenotype may be the result of the loss of many genes giving rise to what is referred to as a 'contiguous gene syndrome'[77]. In the case of disorders such as Down's syndrome, the phenotype may be due to the effect of a small number of genes[78]. Epstein[79] has argued that it may not be a direct effect of a gene or genes located on chromosome 21 but rather the consequence of trisomy 21 on the expression of other genes or due to a nonspecific disruption of development. Increased activity of the enzyme superoxide dismutase is found in Down's syndrome[80], owing to the fact that the gene for this enzyme is located on chromosome 21. This increased activity causes the formation of free hydroxyl radicals which may be the explanation of the apparent premature aging in Down's syndrome[81].

There has been a very substantial number of studies of the cognitive and neuropathological characteristics of children with Down's syndrome[82,83]. Brain weight at birth is not substantially smaller than normal but fails to grow as would be expected, resulting in a small and abnormally shaped brain with a particular impairment of frontal and occipital lobe development, suggesting a failure of neuronal growth[84]. There is evidence of maldevelopment of the cerebrum, cerebellum and portions of the limbic system and it appears as if the later stages of CNS development are arrested[85]. Abnormalities of dendrite formation, a failure of the normal rationalization of the neuronal architecture and reduced numbers of granular and pyramidal cells have also been reported[86–88]. Particularly with the increased life expectancy of people with this syndrome, the observed increased risk of Alzheimer-like neuropathology and the resultant clinical features of dementia have been intensively studied[89]. More recently, the gene for the amyloid precursor protein has also been located on the long arm of chromosome 21[90]. However, the role of raised amyloid expression as a cause for the high rates of Alzheimer's neuropathology in people with Down's syndrome remains a matter of speculation. Recent observations on two other disorders which are associated with chromosomal abnormalities have highlighted two important mechanisms which are associated with a high probability of intellectual impairment. These are the Fragile-X and the Präder–Willi syndromes. The former is an X-linked disorder which may have a population prevalence of 0.75 per 1000 males and 1.8 per 1000 females[91]. The characteristic fragile site on the long arm of the X chromosome (Xq27.3) was first reported by Lubs[92] when chromosomes were cultured in a folate deficient medium. The physical phenotype is primarily characterized by large ears and jaw, and large testes postpubertally. Specific neuropsychological and speech abnormalities have been reported, such as impairment of short-term memory and arithmetic ability, and 'litanic', 'cluttered' and 'jocular' speech[20]. There is also evidence of a decline in intellectual ability in some but not all males with fragile-X syndrome in their teenage years. Hagerman et al.[93] in a longitudinal study of 24 males with the syndrome reported a significant decline in IQ in 7 of the 24 male subjects, primarily due to relatively greater impairments in abstract reasoning and higher symbolic language. Magnetic resonance imaging studies reported finding evidence of decrease in the size of the posterior cerebellar vermis[94] although whether this finding is indicative of pathology has been questioned. Neuropathological studies have reported evidence of dendritic spin abnormalities in the cortex of people with Fragile-X syndrome but no other definite abnormalities[95]. More recently, CGG repeat sequences of DNA have been found at the fragile site close to the putative gene (FMR-1) for Fragile-X syndrome[96–98]. The abnormal sequence increases in length as it passes through generations. The precise reason why this repeat sequence gives rise to mental handicap is unclear although it may alter the methylation pattern of the FMR-1 gene and thus gene expression.

The Präder–Willi syndrome is characterized by severe neonatal hypotonia, short stature, learning disabilities, delayed secondary sexual development and severe obesity consequent upon an insatiable appetite[99]. Over half of those with this syndrome have been found to have a deletion on the proximal part of the long arm of chromosome 15 (15q11–13)[100]. A deletion at this site is also found in cases of a phenotypically different syndrome, Angelman's syndrome[101]. This disorder is characterized by more severe intellectual impairment, markedly impaired language development, ataxic gait and an apparent happy disposition[102]. These two disorders have been shown to demonstrate the phenomenon of 'genomic imprinting'[103], whereby differential expression of genes depends on the sex of the parents from which they were inherited. Whether a person with a chromosome 15 deletion at 15q11–13 has Präder–Willi or Angelman's syndrome depends upon the parental origin of the deleted chromosome. If it is paternal, then Präder–Willi syndrome develops, if maternal Angelman's syndrome. In support of the role of imprinting is the observation that in those cases of Präder–Willi syndrome in which no chromosomal deletion is found there is iso- or heterodisomy of chromosome 15 with both copies of this chromosome being inherited from the mother. Thus, as is the case with a chromosome 15 deletion, the result is that the child has no paternal copies of the genes on chromosome 15[104]. If the maternal copy or copies of specific genes are switched off due to imprinting then no copies of these genes can be expressed. Flint[105] suggests that imprinting is yet another genetic phenomenon which needs to be considered along with traditional Mendelian models of inheritance, polygenic inheritance, penetrance and epistatic effects in understanding the genetics of psychiatric disorders. There has been little study of the neuropathology of Präder–Willi syndrome but it is likely that there is an abnormality of the normal satiety mechanism which results in severe overeating[106] and abnormalities of hypothalamic nuclei have been reported[107].

Environmental risk factors and brain development

The ultimate level of ability and degree to which a person with an intellectual impairment and learning disability is disadvantaged in society may be strongly influenced by a variety of socially determined factors. The environmental risk factors referred to here are those which may have a direct effect on brain development and thus on the future intellectual and emotional development of that person. In this context, although the distinction between genetically and environmentally determined abnormalities of brain development is clearly a useful one, the boundaries can become blurred. For example, babies with genetic disorders have an increased risk of experiencing environmentally determined insults and the extent of any disability following perinatal trauma may depend upon the biological response to such injury. This may be at least partially genetically determined[108].

Specific prenatal environmental risk factors are well known and include maternal infections such as congenital rubella[109], cytomegalovirus[110] and toxoplasmosis[111] infections. More recently congenitally acquired immune deficiency syndrome has been reported to be associated with developmental delay and in three children definite cognitive decline and dementia occurred. In three cases, postmortem examination demonstrated the presence of subacute cytomegalovirus infection, nonspecific white matter changes and calcification within cerebral vasculature of the basal ganglion[112]. These disorders are in essence preventable through public health and vaccination policies. Another potentially preventable disorder is the fetal alcohol syndrome[113]. The effects on the fetus of excessive maternal alcohol consumption including pre- and postnatal growth retardation, craniofacial abnormalities and intellectual impairment of varying degrees[114]. There have been many animal studies and follow-up studies of humans who had been subjected to varying amounts of maternal alcohol consumption when in utero. The findings of studies in humans may be confounded by other effects such as nutritional deficiencies during pregnancy and in early childhood, and psychosocial factors. However, there is now very considerable data showing a major effect on the fetus of significant maternal alcohol consumption. For example, Russell et al.[115] examined the predictive value of specific indicators of maternal alcohol consumption on future childhood development. In their earlier study[116], they reported that the amount of alcohol drunk per day prior to pregnancy was associated with increased spontaneous abortions and lower fetal apgar scores. Measures of problem drinking during pregnancy were associated with small head circumference, lower birth weight and lower apgar scores. The authors followed up 313 children born to mothers who were categorized as follows: abstainers, light/moderate drinkers and heavy or problem drinkers. They were able to include a final sample size of 175 children. As with other studies[117,118], there was evidence of an association between the amount of alcohol consumed by the mother during pregnancy and the presence in the child of dysmorphic features characteristic of the fetal alcohol syndrome, impaired growth, a reduced head circumference and a reduced Verbal IQ. Studies of rat fetuses exposed to alcohol in utero found abnormalities of the hippocampal mossy fibres[119] suggesting abnormality of migration as well as an effect on the shape of the neurones themselves. Postnatal exposure of the rats to alcohol, which is the equivalent to exposure in the last trimester of a human pregnancy, had an even more severe effect. Many other studies have reported abnormalities in the developing neurotransmitter systems of rats exposed to alcohol in utero. For example, Druse et al.[120] describes a deficiency of 5-HT and 5-HIAA in the brain stem and motor cortex. The authors also report a failure of normal developmental decline of these receptors.

The area of environmental risk factors which has received considerable attention is that of fetal damage in the perinatal period secondary to hypoxia or traumatic injury and the relationship of this to the occurrence of cerebral palsy[121]. The proportion of cases of mental handicap which can be attributed to perinatal injury within a population is far from clear. Of people living in institutions 2 studies reported that damage during the perinatal period was the explanation for the handicap in as high as 30% in one study, and as low as 4.0% in another[122-124]. A prevalence study of cerebral palsy reported rates of 3.6 per 1000 in children aged 5 to 14 years of age but the authors estimated that, given the fact that other cases were later identified as a result of a door to door survey, the prevalence rate was nearer 5.8 per 1000[125]. In studies of cerebral palsy, the presence of particular types of motor disabilities in the absence of an identifiable progressive disorder are the main criteria for inclusion, the presence or not of intellectual impairment is not part of the criteria. It is well established that the main predictor of cerebral palsy is birthweight and gestational age (see Fig. 4). Stanley and Alberman[121] in their review discuss the complex relationship between different factors such as birthweight, gestational age, growth rate and measures of fetal immaturity on the relative risk of occurrence of either spastic diplegia or cerebral palsy. The

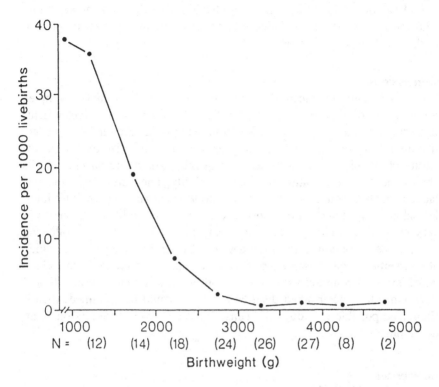

Fig. 4. Diagram of the birth weight specific incidence of cerebral palsy by 500g groups in the years 1973–76. (Taken from Hagberg & Hagberg, 1984 [122].)

crucial issues are prevention through increasingly refined neonatal care and the identification and amelioration of cerebral damage by detection of, for example, cerebral hemorrhage using ultrasound. Roth et al.[126] have used magnetic resonance spectroscopy (MRS) to assess the cerebral oxidative metabolism of babies who have suffered birth asphyxia. In the study 52 infants were included and the 38 surviving infants were assessed neuro-developmentally at 1 year. Evidence of hypoxic–ischaemic damage was found on ultrasound in 27 infants and, in those 14 with severe impairments, there was evidence later of cyst development or ventricular dilation characteristic of loss of brain tissue. Change in the spectra characteristic of a fall in ATP with a failure to rise later indicated a bad prognosis.

More recent epidemiological work has focused on the outcome of babies born with low birthweights. For example, in a report from the Scottish low birthweight study[127], 896 of 908 livebirths weighing less than 1750 g at birth were followed up. At the age of 4.5 years, 71% had survived. Of the 611 of these who were assessed, 16% were disabled, the majority having cerebral palsy. The others had sensory impairments. The authors report a prevalence

A J Holland

rate of cerebral palsy of 52.5 per 1000 livebirths in this population. Those who had weighed less than 1000 g at birth accounted for a greater proportion of those with a severe disability.

Conclusions

The term 'mental handicap' does little justice to what is a highly complex group of disorders which have in common delayed childhood development, impairment in the acquisition of social and living skills and impaired intellectual ability. More recent methods of classification emphasize the interactive nature of the biological substrate, subsequent learning and an individual's environment in the causation of chronic disability. There are many biological factors which undoubtedly affect brain development and thereby limit intellectual attainment and, in the most severe cases, shorten life or can result in very extreme disabilities. There are many points in the process following neural tube formation to the fully developed brain in adolescence at which abnormalities might arise. There may be certain weak points in this chain which are final common pathways for both genetically, chromosomally and environmentally determined disorders. If these could be identified, then it should be possible to reduce the consequences of such disorders on brain development.

References

(1) Clarke AM, Clarke ADB. Constancy and change in the growth of human characteristics. The 1st Jack Tizzard Memorial Lecture. *J Child Psych Psychiat* 1984; 25: 191–210.
(2) Law J, Conway J. Effect of abuse and neglect on the development of children's speech and language. *Dev Med Child Neurol* 1992; 32: 943–8.
(3) Zigler E, Berman W. Discerning the future of early childhood intervention. *Am Psych* 1983; 38: 894–906.
(4) Frith U. Cognitive development and cognitive deficit. *Psychologist* 1992; 5: 13–19.
(5) Rutter M, Graham P, Yule W. *A neuropsychiatric study in childhood.* London: Spastics International Medical Publications, 1970.
(6) Corbett JA. Psychiatric morbidity and mental retardation. In: Snaith P, James FE, eds. *Psychiatric illness in mental handicap.* Ashford: Hedley Brothers, 1979.
(7) Ballinger BR, Reid AH. Psychiatric disorder in an adult training centre and a hospital for the mentally handicapped. *Psych Med* 1977; 7: 525–8.
(8) Lund J. The prevalence of psychiatric morbidity in mentally retarded adults. *Acta Psychiat Scand* 1985; 72: 563–70.
(9) Fryers T. *The epidemiology of severe intellectual impairment: the dynamics of prevalence.* London: Academic Press, 1984.
(10) Shah A, Holmes N, Wing L. Prevalence of autism and related conditions in adults in a mental handicap hospital. *App Res Ment Handicap* 1982; 3: 303–17.
(11) Ellis D. *Sensory impairments in mentally handicapped people.* London: Croom Helm, 1986.

(12) Corbett JA, Harris R, Robinson RG. Epilepsy. In: Wortis J, ed. *Mental retardation and developmental disabilities*. New York: Bruner Mazel, 1975, vol. VII.

(13) *World Health Organization manual of the international statistical classification of diseases, injuries and causes of death*. 8th ed. Geneva: World Health Organization, 1969.

(14) *World Health Organization international classification of impairments, disabilities and handicaps*. Geneva: World Health Organization, 1980.

(15) Fryers T. Epidemiological issues in mental retardation. *J Ment Defic Res* 1987; 31: 365–84.

(16) Hodapp RM, Burack JA, Zigler E. *Issues in the developmental approach to mental retardation*. Cambridge: Cambridge University Press, 1990.

(17) Attwood A, Frith U, Hermelin V. The understanding and use of interpersonal gesture by autistic and Down's syndrome children. *J Autism Dev Disorders* 1988; 18: 251–7.

(18) Cicchetti D, Sroufe LA. The relationship between affective and cognitive developmental in Down syndrome children. *Child Dev* 1976; 47: 920–9.

(19) Hodapp RM, Dykens EM, Hagerman RJ, Schreiner R, Lachiewicz AM, Leckman JF. Developmental implications of changing trajectories of IQ in males with Fragile X syndrome. *J Am Acad Child Adolesc Psychiat* 1990; 29(2): 214–19.

(20) Sudhalter V, Maranion M, Brookes P. Expressive semantic deficit in the productive language of males with Fragile X syndrome. *Am J Med Genet* 1992; 43: 65–71.

(21) Edelman GM. Cell-adhesion molecules: a molecular basis for animal form. *Sci Am* 1984; 250(4): 118–29.

(22) Purves D, Lichtman JW. *Principles of neural development*. Sunderland, Mass: Sinauer Associates Inc., 1985.

(23) Levitt P, Cooper ML, Rakie CP. Co-existence of neuronal and glial precursor cells in the cerebral ventricular zone of the fetal monkey: an ultra structural immunoperoxidase study. *J Neurosci* 1981; 1: 27–39.

(24) White JG, Horvitz RH, Sulston JE. Neuro differentiation in cell lineage mutants of caenorhabditis elegans. *Nature* 1983; 297: 584–7.

(25) Kimble JE. Strategies for control of pattern formation in caernorhabditis elegans. *Phil Trans R Soc Lond (Biol)* 1981; 295: 539–51.

(26) Sulston JE, Horvitz RH. Abnormal cell lineages in mutants of the nematode caenorhabditis elegans. *Dev Biol* 1981; 82: 41–55.

(27) Kriegstein AR, Dichter MA. Morphological classification of rat cortical neurons in cell culture. *J Neurosci* 1983; 3: 1634–47.

(28) Levinthal F, Macagno E, Levinthal C. Anatomy and development of identified cells in isogenic organisms. *Cold Spring Harbor Symp Quant Biol* 1975; 40: 321–33.

(29) Lander AD. Understanding the molecules of neurol cell contacts: emerging patterns of structure and function. *Trends Neurosci* 1989; 12: 189–95.

(30) Gadisseux JF, Kadhim HJ, van den Bosch de Aguilar P, Caviness VS, Evrard P. Neuron migration within the radial glial fiber systems of the developing murine cerebrum: an electron microscopic autoradiographic analysis. *Dev Brain Res* 1990; 52: 39–56.

(31) Levy HL, Waisbren SE. The effects of untreated maternal phenylketonuria and hyperphenylalaninemia on the foetus. *N Eng J Med* 1983; 309: 1269–74.

(32) Miller MW. Effect of prenatal exposure to alcohol on the distribution and time of origin of cortico-spinal neurones in the rat. *J Comp Neurol* 1987; 257: 272–82.

(33) Berg DK. Cell death in neuronal development regulation by trophic factors. In: Spitzer NC, ed. *Neuronal development*. New York: Plenum Press, 1982, 297–331.

(34) Greene LA. Quantitative in vitro studies on the nerve growth factor (NGF) requirement of neurons. II. Sensory neurons. *Dev Biol* 1977; 58: 106–13.

(35) Schwartz JP, Breakfield XP. Altered nerve growth factor in fibroblasts from patients with familial dysautonomia. *Proc Nat Acad Sci USA* 1980; 77: 1154–8.

(36) Gurney ME. Suppression of terminal sprouting at the neuromuscular junction by immune sera. *Nature* 1984; 307: 546–8.

(37) Cowan WM, Fawsett JW, O'Leary DDM, Stanfield BB. Regressive events in neurogenesis. *Science* 1984; 225: 1258–65.

(38) Shatz CJ. Impulse activity and the patterning of connections during CNS development. *Neuron* 1990; 5: 745–56.

(39) Hubel DH, Wiesel TN. The period of susceptibility to the physiological effects of unilateral eye closure in kittens. *J Physiol* 1970; 206: 419–36.

(40) Sherman SM, Spear PD. Organisation of the visual pathways in normal and visually deprived cats. *Physiol Rev* 1982; 62: 738–855.

(41) Shatz CJ. The prenatal development of the cat's retinogeniculate pathway. *J Neurosci* 1983; 3: 482–99.

(42) Hubel DH, Wiesel TN, LeVay S. Plasticity of ocular dominance columns in the monkey striate cortex. *Phil Trans Roy Soc (Lond) B* 1977; 278: 3700–409.

(43) Wiesel TN, Hubel DH. Comparison of the effects on unilateral and bilateral eye closure on cortical unit responses in kittens. *J Neurophysiol* 1965; 28: 1029–40.

(44) Stryker MP, Harris W. Binocular impulse blockade prevents the formation of the ocular dominance columns in cat visual cortex. *J Neurosci* 1986; 6: 2117–33.

(45) Meister M, Wong ROL, Baylor DA, Shatz C. Syndronous bursting activity in ganglion cells of the developing mammalian retina. *Invest Ophth Vis Sci* 1990 (suppl) 31: 115.

(46) Fregnac Y, Schulz D, Thorpe S, Bienenstock E. A cellular analogue of visual cortical plasticity. *Nature* 1988; 333: 367–70.

(47) Brown TH, Kairiss EW, Keenana C. Hevvian synapses: mechanisms and algorithms. *Ann Rev Neurosci* 1990; 13: 475–511.

(48) Huttenlocher PR, de Courten C, Garey LJ, van de Loos H. Synaptogenesis in human visual cortex – evidence for synapse elimination during normal development. *Neurosci Lett* 1982; 33: 247–52.

(49) Takashima S, Chan F, Becker LE, Armstrong DL. Morphology of the developing visual cortex of the human infant: a quantitative and qualitative Golgi study. *J Neuropathol Exp Neurol* 1980; 39: 487–501.

(50) Schade JP, van Groenigne WB. Structural organisation of the human cerebral cortex. I. Maturation of the middle frontal gyrus. *Acta Anat* 1961; 47: 74–111.

(51) Rutter M. Continuities and discontinuities from infancy. In: Osofsky J, ed. *Handbook of infant development* 2nd ed. New York: John Wiley, 1987: 1256–98.

(52) Werker JF, Tees RC. Cross-language speech perception: evidence for perceptual reorganisation during the first year of life. *Inf Behav Dev* 1984; 7: 49–63.

(53) Goodman R. Developmental disorders and structural brain development. In: Rutter M, Casaer P, eds. *Biological risk factors for psychosocial disorders*. Cambridge: Cambridge University Press, 1991.

(54) Harwerth RS, Smith EL, Duncan GC, Crawford MLJ, von Noorden GK. Multiple sensitive periods in the development of the primate visual system. *Science* 1986; 232: 235–8.

(55) Penrose LS. Clinical and genetic study of 1280 cases of mental defect. *Special report series of Medical Research Coun*, vol 229, London: HMSO, 1938.

(56) Geschwind N, Galaburda AM. Cerebral lateralisation biological mechanisms associations and pathology: I. A hypothesis and a programme for research. *Arch Neurol* 1985; 42: 428–59.

(57) Lewis EO. Types of mental deficiency and their social significance. *J Ment Sci* 1933; 79: 298–304.

(58) Tredgold AF. *Mental deficiency*. 8th ed. London: Bailière Tindall, 1952.

(59) Nichols PL. Familial mental retardation. *Behav Genet* 1984; 14: 161–70.

(60) Birch HG, Richardson SA, Baird D, Horobin G, Illsley R. *Mental subnormality in the community: a clinical epidemiological study*. Baltimore, Maryland: Williams and Wilkins, 1970.

(61) Clarke AM, Clarke ADB, Berg JM. *Mental deficiency: the changing outlook*. 4th ed. London: Methuen, 1985.

(62) Hagberg B, Hagberg G. Aspects of prevention of pre, peri and postnatal brain pathology in severe and mild mental retardation and analysis from recent Swedish epidemiological research. In: Dobbing J, Clarke ADB, Corbett J et al., eds. *Scientific studies in mental retardation*. London: Royal Society of Medicine, 1984.

(63) Watts RWE, Gibbs DA. *Lysosomal storage diseases: biochemical and clinical aspects*. London: Taylor and Francis, 1986.

(64) Stern J. The biochemical approach to mental handicap: 30 years of achievements and disappointments. *J Ment Defic Res* 1987; 31: 357–64.

(65) Wahlstrom J. Gene map of mental retardation. *J Ment Defic Res* 1990; 34: 11–27.

(66) Cowie VA. Phenylpyruvic oligophrenia. *J Ment Sci* 1951; 97: 505–31.

(67) Hudson FP, Mordaunt VL, Leahy I. Evaluation of treatment begun in first three months of life in 184 cases of phenylketonuria. *Arch Dis Childh* 1970; 45: 5–12.

(68) Brunner RL, Berch DB, Berry H. PKU and complex spacial visualisation. *Dev Med Child Neurol* 1987; 29: 460–8.

(69) Lou HC, Lykklund AM, Udesen H, Brunhn P. Increased vigilance and dopamine synthesis by large doses of tyrosine or phenylalanine restriction in phenylketonuria. *Acta Pediat Scand* 1987; 76: 560–5.

(70) Harkness RA, Pollitt RJ, Addison GM. Inborn errors of cellular organelles. *J Inherited Metab Dis* 1987; 10(suppl): 1–220.

(71) Levan A. Chromosome studies in some human tumours and tissues of normal origin, grown in vivo and in vitro at the Sloan–Kettering Institute. *Cancer* 1956; 9: 648–63.

(72) Jacobs PA. Review: the role of chromosome abnormalities in reproductive failure. *Reprod Nutr Dev 1990; (Suppl 1): 63s–74s.*

(73) Wilkie AOM, Buckle VJ, Harris PC et al. Clinical features and molecular analysis of the a-thalassemia/mental retardation syndromes. I. Cases due to deletions involving chromosome band 16p13.3. *Am J Hum Genet* 1990; 46: 1112–26.

(74) Lamb J, Harris PC, Lindenbaum RH et al. Detection of breakpoints in submicroscopic chromosomal translocation, illustrating an important mechanism for genetic disease. *Lancet* ii 1989; 819–24.

(75) Chandley AC. Asymmetry in chromosome pairing: a major factor in de novo mutation and the production of genetic disease in man. *J Med Genet* 1989; 26: 546–52.

(76) Ferguson-Smith MA. Invited editorial: putting the genetics back into cytogenetics. *Am J Hum Genet* 1991; 48: 179–82.

(77) Schmickel RD. Contiguous gene syndromes: a component of recognisable syndromes. *J Paedia* 1986; 109: 231–41.

(78) Opitz JM, Gibert-Barness EF. Reflections on the pathogenesis of Down's syndrome. *Am J Med Genet* 1990; (suppl 7): 38–51.

(79) Epstein CJ. The consequences of chromosome inbalance. *Am J Med Genet* 1990; (suppl 7): 31–7.

(80) Brooksbank VWL, Balazs R. Superoxide dismutase and lipoperoxidation in Down's syndrome fetal brain. *Lancet* 1983; i: 881–2.

(81) Martin GM. Genetic syndrome in man with potential relevance to the pathobiology of ageing. In: Bergsma D, Harrison DE, Paul NW, eds. *Genetic effects on ageing, birth defects, original article series.* New York: The National Foundation – March of Dimes/A R Liss, 1978: 5–39.

(82) Nadel L. *The psychobiology of Down syndrome.* Cambridge, Mass: MIT Press, 1988.

(83) Cicchetti D, Beeghly M. *Children with Down syndrome: a developmental perspective.* Cambridge: Cambridge University Press, 1990.

(84) Benda CE. Mongolism. In: Mencken J, ed. *Pathology of the nervous system.* 1971; vol 2: 1361–71.

(85) Courchesne E. Physioanatomical considerations in Down syndrome. In: Nadel L, ed. *The psychobiology of Down syndrome.* Cambridge, Mass: MIT Press, 1988.

(86) Wisniewski K, Laure-Kaminowska M, Connell F, Wen G. Neuronal density and synaptogenesis in the postnatal stage of brain maturation in Down syndrome. In: Epstein CJ, ed. *The neurobiology of Down syndrome.* New York: Raven Press, 1986: 29–44.

(87) McGram-Hill, Wisniewski KE, Laure-Kaminowska M, Wisniewski HM. Evidence of arrest of neurogenesis and synaptogenesis in brains of patients with Down's syndrome. *N Eng J Med* 1984; 311: 1187–8.

(88) Kemper TL. Neuropathology of Down syndrome. In: Nadel L, ed. *The psychobiology of Down syndrome.* National Down's Syndrome Society, 1988.

(89) Oliver C, Holland AJ. Down's syndrome and Alzheimer's disease: a review. *Psychol Med* 1986; 16: 307–22.

(90) Goldgaber D, Lerman MI, MacBride OW, Saffioti U, Gajdusecek DC. Charac-

terisation and chromosomal localisation of a cDNA encoding brain amyloid of Alzheimer's disease. *Science* 1987; 235: 877–80.

(91) Webb TP, Bundey S, Thake A, Todd J. The frequency of the Fragile X chromosome among school children in Coventry. *J Med Genet* 1986; 23: 396–9.

(92) Lubs HA. A marker X chromosome. *Am J Hum Genet* 1969; 21: 231–44.

(93) Hagerman RJ, Schreiner RA, Kemper MB, Wittenberger MD, Zahn B, Habicht K. Longitudinal IQ changes in fragile X males. *Am J Med Genet* 1989; 33: 513–18.

(94) Reiss AL, Alyward E, Freund L, Joshi PK, Bryan RN. Neuroanatomy of Fragile X syndrome: the posterior fossa. *Ann Neurol* 1991; 29: 26–32.

(95) Hinton VJ, Brown WT, Wisniewski K, Rudelli RD. Analysis of Neocortex in three males with the fragile X syndrome. *Am J Med Genet* 1991; 41: 289–94.

(96) Rousseau F, Heitz D, Biancalana V et al. Direct diagnosis by DNA analysis of the Fragile X syndrome of mental retardation. *N Eng J Med* 1991; 325: 1673–81.

(97) Verker KA, Pieretti M, Sutcliffe J et al. Identification of a gene (FMR-1) containing a CGG repeat coincident with a break point cluster region exhibiting length variation in Fragile X syndrome. *Cell* 1991; 65: 905–14.

(98) Yu S, Pritchard M, Kremer E et al. Fragile X geneo-type characterised by an unstable region of DNA. *Science* 1991; 252: 1179–81.

(99) Laurance BM. Hypotonia, mental retardation, obesity and cryptorchidism associated with dwarfism and diabetes in children. *Arch Dis Childh* 1967; 42: 126–39.

(100) Ledbetter DH, Riccardi VM, Airhart SD et al. Deletions of chromosome 15 as a cause of Präder–Willi syndrome. *N Eng J Med* 1981; 304: 325–8.

(101) Williams CA, Gray BA, Hendrickson JE et al. Incidence of 15q deletions in the Angelman syndrome: a survey of twelve affected persons. *Am J Med Genet* 1989; 32: 339–45.

(102) Angelman H. 'Puppet' children: a report on three cases. *Dev Med Child Neurol* 1965; 7: 681–8.

(103) Hall JG. Genomic imprinting: a review and relevance to human disease. *Am J Hum Genet* 1990; 46: 857–73.

(104) Nichols RD, Knoll JHM, Butler MF, Karam S, Lalande M. Genetic imprinting suggested by maternal heterodisomy in non-deletion Präder–Willi syndrome. *Nature* 1989; 342: 281–5.

(105) Flint J. Implications of genomic imprinting for psychiatric genetics. *Psychol Med* 1992; 22: 5–10.

(106) Holland AJ, Treasure J, Coskeran P, Dallow J, Milton N, Hillhouse E. Measurement of excessive appetite and metabolic changes in Präder–Willi syndrome. *Int J Obesity* (in press).

(107) Swaab DF, Roozendaal B, Ravid R, Vellis DN, Gooren L, Williams RS. Suprachiasmatic nucleus in aging, Alzheimer's disease, transsexuality and Präder–Willi syndrome. In: de Kloet ER, Wiegant VM, de Wied D, eds. *Neuropeptides and brain function. Progress in Brain Research* 1987; 72: 301–10.

(108) Berg JM. Physical determinants of environmental origin. In: Clarke AM, Clarke ADB, Berg JM, eds. *Mental deficiency the changing outlook*. London: Methuen, 1985.

(109) Miller K, Craddocik-Watson JE, Pollock TM. Consequences of confirmed maternal rubella at successive stages of pregnancy. *Lancet* 1982; ii: 781–4.

(110) Reynolds DW, Stagno S, Stubbs KG et al. Inapparent congenital cytomegalovirus infection and elevated cord IgM levels: causal relation with auditory and mental deficiency. *N Eng J Med* 1974; 290: 291–6.

(111) Wilson CB, Remington JS, Stagno S, Reynolds DW. Development of adverse sequeoilae in children born with sub-clinical congenital toxoplasma infection. *Pediatrics* 19980; 66: 764–74.

(112) Belman AL, Ultmann MH, Horoupian D et al. Neurological complications in infants and children with acquired immune deficiency syndrome. *Ann Neurol* 1985; 18(5): 560–6.

(113) Jones K, Smith DW. Recognition of a fetal alcohol syndrome in early infancy. *Lancet* 1973; ii: 999–1001.

(114) Porter R. Mechanisms of alcohol damage in utero. Ciba Foundation Symposium 105. London: Pitman, 1984.

(115) Russell M, Czarnecki DM, Cowan R, McPherson E, Mudar PJ. Measures of maternal alcohol use as predictors of development in early childhood. *Alcoholism: Clin Exp Res* 1991; 15(6): 991–1000.

(116) Russell M, Skinner JB. Early measure of maternal alcohol misuse as predictors of adverse pregnancy outcomes. *Alcoholism* 1988; 12(6): 824–30.

(117) Streissguth AP, Aase JM, Clarren SK et al. Fetal alcohol syndrome in adolescents and adults. *J Am Med Assn* 1991; 265(15): 1961–7.

(118) Spohr HL, Steinhausen HC. Follow-up studies of children with fetal alcohol syndrome. *Neuropediatrics* 1987; 18: 13–17.

(119) West JR, Dewey SL, Pierce DR, Black Jnr AC. Prenatal and early postnatal exposure to ethanol permanently alters the rate hippocampus. In: *Mechanisms of alcohol damage in utero. Ciba Foundation Symposium 105.* London: Pitman, 1984: 8–25.

(120) Druse MJ, Kuo A, Tajuddin N. Effects of in utero ethanol exposure on the developing serotonergic system. *Alcohol* 1991; 15(4): 678–84.

(121) Stanley F, Alberman E, eds. *The epidemiology of the cerebral palsies.* London: Spastics International Medical Publications, 1984.

(122) Hagberg B, Hagberg G. Prenatal and perinatal risk factors in a survey of 681 Swedish cases. In: Stanley F, Alberman E, eds. *The epidemiology of the cerebral palsies. Clinical and Developmental Medicine No. 87.* Spastics International Medical Publications. Oxford: Blackwell, 1984.

(123) Czeizel A, Lany-Engellmayer A, Klujber L, Metneki J, Tusnady G. Aetiological study of mental retardation in Budapest, Hungary. *Am J Ment Defic* 1980; 85: 120–8.

(124) Hunter AGW, Evans JA, Thompson DR, Ramsay S. A study of institutionalised mentally retarded patients in Manatoba. 1. Classification and preventability. *Dev Med Child Neurol* 1980; 22: 145–62.

(125) Levin ML, Brightman IJ, Burtt EJ. The problems of cerebral palsy. *NY State J Med* 1949; 49: 2793–9.

(126) Roth SC, Edwards AD, Cady EB et al. Relation between cerebral oxidative metabolism following birth asphyxia and neurodevelopmental outcome and brain growth. *Dev Med Child Neurol* 1992; 34(4): 285–95.

(127) The Scottish Low Birthweight Study Group. The Scottish low birthweight study: I. Survival, growth, neuromotor and sensory impairment. *Arch Dis Childh* 1992; 67: 675–81.

HIV infection and the brain: an examination of clinical and pathological effects

I P EVERALL and P L LANTOS

Introduction

The recognition of acquired immune deficiency syndrome (AIDS) began in 1981 with the first case reports describing pneumocystis pneumonia and Kaposi's sarcoma in young homosexual men in the United States[1,2]. It was not until at least 2 years later that involvement of the nervous system was realized with the clinical recognition of neurological disorders in up to 50% of patients with AIDS[3]. Over the ensuing decade, from 1981, there has been identification of the causative organism, the human immune deficiency virus[4,5] (HIV), and an increasing understanding of both the characteristics of this virus and its effects on the central nervous system. Clinically, one of the commonest organic neuropsychiatric complications is a dementia, variously named, that occurs in patients with AIDS[6]. This dementing illness is thought to be due directly to HIV infection in the brain.

In this chapter, the following issues will be addressed: first, the characteristics of the virus itself including neurotropic strains and entry into the central nervous system (CNS); secondly, neuropsychological and neuroimaging findings both in the asymptomatic individual and the ill patient, and thirdly, neuropathological findings, their possible evolution, and the correlation of neuropathology and clinical dementia. Finally, neuronal loss and the potential mechanisms for neurotoxicity will be discussed. For a review of opportunistic infections and neoplasms see Everall and Lantos[7].

Viral characteristics

Molecular features

HIV, is one of the retroviruses, which are characterized by containing a single stranded RNA genome with an RNA-dependent DNA polymerase. Entry

All correspondence to: Dr I P Everall, Department of Neuropathology, Institute of Psychiatry, De Crespigny Park, London SE5 8AF, UK

Cambridge Medical Reviews: Neurobiology and Psychiatry Volume 2
© Cambridge University Press

into host cells requires attachment of the virus to a cell surface receptor. Initially, the CD4 molecule was thought to be essential for a cell to be susceptible to infection by HIV[8,9], as the primary target of infection was originally identified as CD4 bearing, T-helper lymphocytes[10]. However, the virus has subsequently been identified in other cells, such as macrophages[11] and postulated modes of entry into these cells include attachment of a non-neutralizing antibody to the virus, with the subsequent virus–antibody complex being brought into contact with cells by attachment of the antibody to either a host cell membrane complement or Fc receptor[12,13].

Following attachment, the viral RNA genome enters the host cell together with the reverse transcriptase which synthesizes a double stranded DNA copy of the viral genome. This DNA copy enters the nucleus where it becomes integrated into the host chromosomes and thus persistently infects the cell. The integrated copy of the viral genome is called a provirus, these genes can replicate along with the host chromosomal DNA and will persist for the life of the cell. During this time, the HIV infection is latent.

The molecular structure of the HIV genome includes three structural genes: *gag*, *env* and *pol*. In addition, there are 7 other genes: *tat*, *rev*, *nef*, *vif*, *vpr*, *vpu* and *vpx*. The first 3 of these additional genes are known to regulate expression of the viral genome; the *tat* gene stimulates, and is essential to, the replication of HIV[14], while the *rev* gene increases the efficiency of replication: deletions in this gene are lethal to the virus[15]. The *nef* gene product is thought to repress replication[16], while the *vif* gene affects viral spread throughout a cell population. HIV strains without the *vif* gene are 100 to 1000 times less infectious[17]. The roles of *vpr*, *vpu* and *vpx* are unclear; the last gene is only found in HIV-2[15].

Regulation of HIV expression within the host cell may be controlled at two levels: first, by the virus itself through regulatory genes, as described above, or secondly, by cellular factors. Cellular factors include the state of the cell. If HIV gains entry to a quiescent T-lymphocyte full viral integration and formation of the provirus may be delayed, whereas when the cell is stimulated DNA synthesis is allowed to proceed, and return to a quiescent state may again halt the activity of reverse transcriptase[18]. The mechanism of this regulation is not known and is confused by the fact that the level of transcription factors and other proteins, which act on the long terminal repeat sequences found at each end of the viral genome, also regulate virus replication[19,20].

In addition, coinfection of the host cell by other infectious agents has been shown to enhance HIV expression, possibly by a mechanism similar to the *tat* gene. These include cytomegalovirus, mycoplasma[21,22] and the human herpes virus-6[23]. Even in the brain coinfection of HIV infected cells by other viruses, including the JC virus[24], can result in activation of HIV replication and a more severe HIV encephalitis.

HIV variability

It is known that HIV is variable in its genome sequence between different isolates, either from different individuals or from the same individual at different stages of the disease[25,26]. Some regions of the genome remain conserved while others, especially the *env* region, are very variable[27]. This variation is thought to be important for pathogenesis of AIDS as the variants of the virus isolated later from an individual, when they have become unwell, demonstrate the following characteristics that are thought to be associated with virulence[16]:

a) increased cellular host range,
b) more rapid replication,
c) high titres of virus in infected cells,
d) altered cell membrane permeability causing increased entry of monovalent and divalent cations, along with water,
e) efficient cell killing probably due to the fusion and ballooning of infected cells resulting from the membrane changes,
f) greater affinity for nonneutralizing antibodies (hence increasing the probability of infecting non-CD4+ cells), and
g) escape from the suppressive effect on replication by the *nef* gene product, hence accelerating replication.

The genomic variation not only produces more virulent strains but there is diversity in tropism, including the emergence of neurotropic strains. Neurotropism refers to the predilection of the virus for nervous tissue and maybe accompanied by neurotoxicity, that is destruction of neurones and other nervous tissue. These strains differ in preferentially replicating in monocytes and macrophages, whereas blood isolates have a preference for T-cells[28,29]. The preference for monocytes and macrophages form the main reservoir of the virus in the brain. The development of neurotropism is thought to be linked to alterations in the envelope glycoprotein gp120, as a single amino acid change in the CD4 binding domain has been shown to determine cellular tropism[30]. The neurotropic variants that infect monocytes, microglia, macrophages, and macrophage derived multinucleated giant cells are found in levels of between 500 and 1500 copies of HIV RNA per cell, which is 10 times higher than in peripheral leucocytes[31].

Entry into the CNS

There are two issues to be clarified when considering entry into the CNS. First, how HIV enters into the brain, and secondly, at what stage is the brain infected. This latter point is important in ascribing early neurological features to HIV. Currently, it is known that a few weeks after infection, clinically a self-limiting aseptic meningitis may occur. HIV antigen has been isolated from the CSF at this time[32]. The brain thus appears to be an early target for infection, although the infected individual remains asymptomatic apart from early subtle cognitive deficits which may occur.

The mode of entry of the virus into the brain remains less clear, but there are a number of possible mechanisms. Most studies suggest that bone marrow derived, HIV infected, monocytes transport the virus into the brain as they migrate from the systemic circulation into the brain. This is the Trojan horse theory[33]. Additionally, there is evidence that activated T-cells can enter the CNS, thus raising the possibility that these cells can introduce HIV into the brain. According to alternative hypotheses free virus may enter and replicate either in vascular endothelium[34] or choroid plexus cells[35] or the virus gains entrance via peripheral nerves. However, these latter observations as a route of brain infection are disputed.

There remains some doubt as to which cells within the brain are vulnerable to infection by HIV. A number of reports, utilizing a range of techniques, including electron microscopy, immunocytochemistry and in situ hybridization, have detected viral particles in astrocytes[34,36], oligodendrocytes and neurons[37,38]. The significance of these findings remains to be established, as the positive findings occurred in isolated cases, cell specific markers were not used to identify definitively the cell, and the results have not been confirmed by other investigators. Currently, there is no substantive evidence to support infection of any neuroectodermal cells[39] and it is assumed that monocytes, macrophages and multinucleated giant cells are the only cells to be infected by, and contain HIV in the brain.

Clinical findings

As early as 1983, neurological abnormalities were recognized as important complications that can affect over 50% of patients[3]. These abnormalities include motor and sensory peripheral neuropathies, myelopathies, and most importantly a dementing illness, that can be both severe and rapid in its progress, and is thought to be due directly to HIV. There is as yet no definite evidence that HIV induces psychotic illness, although such illnesses do occur in patients infected with HIV[40]. This chapter will concentrate on HIV dementia.

Clinical features

The clinical features, characterization and even nomenclature of the dementia associated with HIV infection are still being elucidated. It was first described in 1986[41] and was termed AIDS dementia complex to denote the constellation of both cognitive and motor abnormalities that were assumed to coexist as part of the same disease process. The motor symptoms ranged from very mild clumsiness to paraparesis or paraplegia and double incontinence[6]. The cognitive abnormalities commenced with an increasing tendency to be forgetful but insufficient to interfere with the activities of daily living. Over time, the cognitive deficits increased in severity to prevent independent living and finally to progress to a mute vegetative state. The prognosis was extremely poor with death occurring in 4 to 6 months after the onset of severe dementia[6]. Unfortunately, the staging scheme proposed[42], 4 stages from normal, through mild, moderate and severe, to end stage, gave equal importance to motor and cognitive abnormalities. Therefore, even in the absence of cognitive abnormalities, it was possible to rate a patient as suffering from severe dementia solely on account of the major motor disability. This confusing misuse of the concept of dementia is now being addressed by the American Academy of Neurology AIDS Task Force[43]. They suggest a more coherent terminology and operational criteria for the diagnosis of HIV-1 associated cognitive/motor complex. This overall complex is split into two levels, according to severity. The first level consists of the mild manifestation group, called HIV-1 associated minor cognitive/motor disorder, where only the most demanding activities of daily living are mildly impaired. The second level is the severe manifestations and consists of two broad disorders, HIV-1 associated dementia complex and HIV-1 associated myelopathy. The latter term is for those patients whose motor or myelopathic dysfunction is more prominent than any cognitive dysfunction. The former term, the HIV-1 associated dementia complex, is subdivided in order to allow for the clinical variability. Thus the disturbances in cognitive, behavioural or motor areas, are subdivided into HIV-1 associated dementia complex (motor) for those with cognitive and motor impairment but no behavioural change, while HIV-1 associated dementia complex (behaviour) refers to patients with cognitive and behavioural abnormalities. If all three domains are present, then no subcategory is necessary. Finally, the classification allows for probable and possible categories, the latter for those cases where the diagnosis cannot be made with certainty as a result of other causes such as opportunistic infections.

There has also been recognition and clarification of the dementia that can affect children infected with HIV. In the same proposed classification[43] this is termed HIV-1 associated progressive encephalopathy of childhood. Affected young children usually fail to acquire, or begin to lose previously established, developmental milestones. In addition, there is often microcephaly. Older children and adolescents may have more recognizable cognitive impairments, such as deteriorating performance at school. All children often have motor symptoms and signs including weakness, spasticity, hyperreflexia, and ataxia. Neuroimaging (CT and MRI) may reveal cerebral atrophy and, in young children, bilateral calcification of the basal ganglia[44]. The prognosis is, as with the adult equivalent, very poor, with progress to severe mental impairment and spastic quadriparesis.

Neuropsychological findings
Following the first report[3] of neurological complications, including dementia, there have been a number of studies attempting to elucidate the characteristics of cognitive impairments and to clarify the stage when they become

manifest. The neuropsychological tests noted to be most affected in patients with HIV dementia include fine motor control (grooved pegboard and finger tapping tests), rapid sequential problem solving (trail making and digit–symbol tests), spontaneity (verbal fluency), visuospatial problem solving (block design test), and visual memory (visual perception)[45].

It remains far from clear the order in which these impairments evolve and when they become clinically significant. Grant et al.[46] in a small study of 16 HIV infected asymptomatic individuals reported that over half of them had cognitive impairments, in that they demonstrated difficulties on at least 2 tests, compared to only 1 out of 11 seronegative individuals. Despite the size of the study, it received media attention and resulted in disruption in the lives of a number of people with HIV infection. There were recommendations for compulsory HIV testing, especially for people with occupations requiring manual dexterity or mental concentration, and military personnel infected with HIV (around 3500–4000 individuals) were removed from stressful or sensitive jobs[47]. A similar small study of 18 HIV infected but otherwise healthy individuals[48] again reported mild abnormalities in the areas of language, attention, visual and auditory information processing, psychomotor speed and memory.

However, these findings were not borne out by two large-scale cohort studies. In the first study, Janssen et al.[49] studied 100 HIV infected homosexual/bisexual individuals from the San Francisco area. The study excluded any individuals with complicating factors such as head injury, drug misuse, learning difficulties, or those over 50 years of age. No differences were observed between this group and an HIV seronegative group. The only impairment to emerge was in 26 individuals with AIDS related complex. The second study was a multicentre investigation[50] of 270 HIV infected homosexual/bisexual individuals and 193 seronegative subjects. Again, no difference was found between the two groups. From these studies, it is concluded that the prevalence of HIV dementia, amongst healthy individuals infected with HIV, is very low, and when neuropsychological abnormalities are found they are often subclinical and their presence does not predict progression to clinical dementia[51].

Neuroimaging findings

Brain pathology can be detected using computerized tomographic scans (CT)[52], but the sensitivity of magnetic resonance imaging (MRI) scans is superior[53]. MRI scans of patients with AIDS reveal abnormalities such as enlargement of cortical sulci and ventricles, and lesions in the white matter[54]. These abnormalities have also been noted in asymptomatic HIV infected and HIV seronegative homosexual individuals[55]. Sonnerborg et al.[56] found that more brain lesions occurred in individuals with AIDS, and that enlargement of the sulci and ventricles may occur later when symptomatic disease commences. In addition, while some brain lesions were found in both HIV infected asymptomatic and HIV seronegative homosexual individuals, they did not occur in a heterosexual control group. McArthur[50], reporting similar findings in the homosexual group, concluded that care must be taken in interpreting the white matter lesions in asymptomatic individuals as they were not related to neurological or neuropsychological abnormalities, and must not be assumed to be indicative of HIV involvement of the brain.

Investigations have not only concentrated on clarifying structural abnormalities, but also have attempted to define functional brain abnormalities in vivo. There are 3 neuroimaging techniques capable of providing information regarding the functional state of the brain: magnetic resonance spectroscopy (MRS), single photon emission computed tomography (SPECT), and positron emission tomography (PET). All have reported abnormal findings in individuals infected with HIV and patients with AIDS.

An in vivo ^{31}P MRS study, which detects adenosine triphosphate (ATP), phosphocreatine (PCr), and inorganic phosphate (Pi), demonstrated that the ratio of ATP/Pi was reduced in HIV infected individuals when compared to controls[57]. The ratio of ATP/Pi reflects the energy state of a cell. This decreased ratio, together with a decreased ratio of PCr/Pi, was more marked when cognitive impairments were present. In addition, even though these abnormalities were present in volumes sampled from the cortical grey and adjacent white matter, they were not present in subcortical grey structures. Another study, using proton MRS, examined the right parietal region in two patients with AIDS. Although MRI had shown no abnormality in this area, decreased levels of N-acetyl aspartate (NAA) were detected by MRS[58]. NAA is considered to be specific to neurons[59] and a decrease in its level is implied to indicate neuronal loss. These findings are important as they demonstrate that MRS is capable of finding abnormalities, including possible neuronal loss, in areas not identified by structural imaging.

Similarly, SPECT studies have identified extensive cortical blood flow abnormalities in patients with AIDS. These include hypoperfusion in the cerebellum and in the cerebral cortex, greatest in the frontal and parietal areas[60]. The extent of this cortical hypoperfusion also correlated with the severity of the cognitive impairments. In contrast to the findings by proton MRS, Kuni et al.[61] reported abnormalities in the basal ganglia by SPECT, which also appeared to correlate with the severity of the dementia. Similar findings of cortical and subcortical perfusion abnormalities, even in patients with cognitive impairments when the MRI is negative, are observed with PET[62]. It appears that SPECT investigations are also sensitive in discerning occasional subtle blood flow abnormalities in asymptomatic HIV infected individuals[63]. This indicates that HIV associated alterations occur at an early stage after infection even though their clinical relevance is unclear.

Neuropathology of HIV infection

Since the mid-1980s, postmortem studies have been undertaken to identify and clarify those lesions in the brain specifically induced by HIV. These primary abnormalities are distinct from secondary brain lesions, such as opportunistic infections and neoplasms, which are indicative of AIDS. Initially, a number of different terms were applied to the putative HIV pathology, for example, subacute encephalitis, AIDS encephalitis, and HIV encephalopathy. However, the precise meanings of these terms were unclear and often did not correlate with clinical findings. Currently, the following terminology has been adopted for the central nervous system disorders of the various manifestations of HIV induced brain lesions. This nomenclature is solely pathological and does not imply clinical correlates at present[64].

HIV encephalitis Often the brain may appear normal on gross examination and the typical features are microscopic. These include multiple foci of inflammatory cells (Fig. 1(a)), including macrophages, microglia and multinucleated giant cells (MGC). The MGCs are thought to occur through the fusion of macrophages (Fig. 1(b),(c)), and they are the histological hallmark of HIV encephalitis. Within MGCs HIV antigen and nucleic acids can be detected by immunocytochemistry[65] and in situ hybridization[34]. The encephalitic lesions are distributed throughout the white matter, basal ganglia, brainstem and cerebral cortex[66]. In addition, there may be microglial nodules which are denser than HIV foci and contain more lymphocytes and rod shaped microglia. As many as 50% of the microglial nodules may be due to opportunistic infection, usually cytomegalovirus and, less commonly, toxoplasmosis[67]. Occasionally, the brain parenchyma including myelinated fibres may be damaged and there is now evidence of neuronal loss[68], previously unnoticed in earlier qualitative descriptive studies. This feature will be discussed later.

HIV leukoencephalopathy There is diffuse damage to the white matter involving myelin loss, reactive astrocytosis, macrophages and multinucleated giant cells[69]. The white matter in the cerebral hemispheres is affected symmetrically and the cerebellar white matter may also be affected. Together with the myelin loss, there is preliminary evidence that the axonal diameter is reduced[70]. Myelin pallor is a term which has previously been applied to the white matter damage, but essentially it refers to paleness of the white matter on myelin stained sections. It may result from white matter damage but may be caused by autolysis or improper staining techniques, thus myelin pallor should not be used synonymously with HIV leukoencephalopathy.

In HIV leukoencephalopathy there is also evidence of alteration in the microcirculation and possible damage to the blood–brain barrier. Small vessels in the white matter demonstrate mural thickening and there are iron

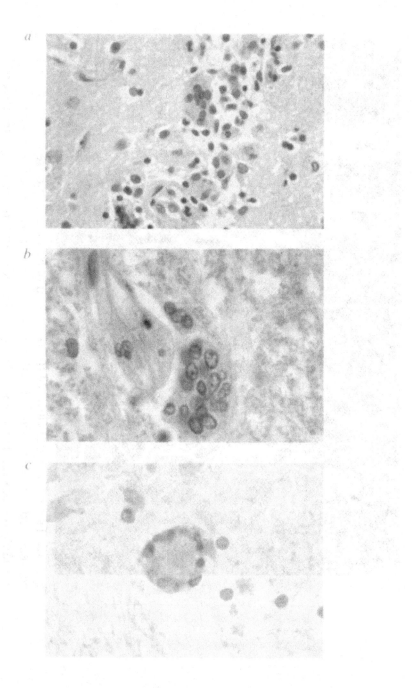

Fig. 1 (*a*). HIV encephalitis. Comprises a collection of inflammatory cells, including multinucleated giant cells, microglial cells and macrophages. Haematoxylin and eosin, × 400.

Figs. (*b*) and (*c*). Multinucleated giant cells, the hallmark of HIV encephalitis. Haematoxylin and eosin, × 800.

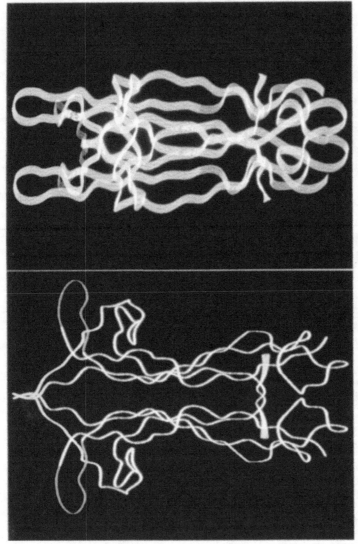

Fig. 12. Two orthogonal views of the α-carbon backbone of mouse β-NGF represented in ribbon form using the program Insight (Biosym Technologies). Variable regions II, III and IV are coloured yellow, green and red, respectively. X-ray coordinates were kindly supplied by Dr J Murray-Rust, Birkbeck College, London. (See p.132.)

deposits, presumably from red blood cells, in perivascular macrophages and multinucleated giant cells[71].

The concept of HIV encephalitis and HIV leukoencephalopathy as two separate entities, while nosologically convenient is still doubtful as they have overlapping features, and in some cases both types of pathology coexist. The frequency of these two diseases is reported as 11% for HIV encephalitis, with an additional 13% having HIV encephalitis and HIV leukoencephalopathy[66].

Vacuolar myelopathy This is a disorder of the spinal cord, predominantly in the dorsolateral spinal tracts. It is characterized by multiple areas with vacuolar myelin swellings and macrophages. The lesions are similar to those of subacute combined degeneration of the cord[72]. Clinically, it may be associated with HIV induced myelopathy.

Vacuolar leukoencephalopathy This is a rare condition with either multifocal or diffuse lesions affecting the white matter in the cerebral hemispheres, cerebellum, basal ganglia or brainstem. There are numerous myelin swellings and macrophages. The features of this condition may also be present in HIV leukoencephalopathy.

Lymphocytic meningitis This condition may be associated with the aseptic meningitis that occurs early after HIV infection. The leptomeninges, including the perivascular spaces, are infiltrated by lymphocytes, but no obvious opportunistic pathogen can be detected.

Diffuse poliodystrophy This term is still controversial as to whether it is a separate entity. Characteristically there is diffuse reactive astrocytosis, gliosis, microglial activation, and possibly neuronal loss in the grey matter of the cerebral cortex, basal ganglia and brainstem nuclei[73].

Cerebral vasculitis including granulomatous angiitis In the walls of cerebral blood vessels, infiltrations of lymphocytes with multinucleated giant cells are found. There may also be accompanying necrosis. It is postulated that this disorder may result in focal neurological deficits.

Early neuropathological changes
The HIV induced CNS lesions outlined above represent fully evolved pathology as the brain is examined postmortem and death results usually from advanced HIV disease. However, it is known that the CNS is infected early on[32]. To date, our understanding of early developing pathology is limited to a few isolated cases where asymptomatic HIV infected individuals died of unrelated causes[74–77]. The findings, in these 'early' cases are nonspecific, including astrocytosis, microglial proliferation, some perivascular cuffing

by inflammatory cells, mild chronic leptomeningitis and, in patients with hemophilia, hemorrhages and infarcts. These findings infer that, while HIV induced CNS pathology may commence at an early asymptomatic stage, HIV encephalitis or leukoencephalopathy may represent more advanced stages in the evolution of HIV induced brain disease.

Clinico-neuropathological correlations

To date, the relationship of the HIV induced neuropathological entities to clinical syndromes is not known. Such understanding of this important question would only be achieved by intensive neurological and neuropsychological investigations of a cohort of patients over a prolonged period of time followed, after death, by a neuropathological examination of the brain. The largest such study[41,78] was undertaken to identify HIV neuropathology and then to correlate this retrospectively with the clinical case notes. The study concluded that, despite variability in both the clinical features and the neuropathology, there seemed to be a correlation between the severity of clinical dementia and the number of multinucleated giant cells and microglial nodules, ie with HIV encephalitis. Further support to this notion was provided by Price et al.[79] who pooled results from earlier smaller studies, and again found that in all those patients who died of severe AIDS dementia there were multinucleated giant cells, and that their number decreased dramatically with only mild or no dementia. However, the observations were made in different sets of patients, and only a quarter to one-half of those investigated had postmortem examination. Therefore, these results can only be considered with some reservation. Similarly, cerebral atrophy, with enlargement of the sulci and ventricles, has been demonstrated by both computer-assisted tomography and magnetic resonance imaging, in HIV dementia[80]. However, the relationship to neuropathological abnormalities is unclear as these changes seem less obvious during postmortem brain examination[42]. Until the association between HIV related brain lesions, neuroimaging, and clinical features is clarified, it has to be assumed that HIV encephalitis, HIV leukoencephalopathy, vacuolar leukoencephalopathy, and diffuse poliodystrophy may all contribute to HIV dementia[66]. Alternatively, the inflammatory changes may not be causal and the dementia may, in fact, be related to neuronal loss, which is now becoming recognized as a feature of HIV infection.

HIV induced neuronal loss and its possible causes

Quantitative studies of HIV Induced CNS pathology

Despite the severe clinical dementia that may complicate HIV infection, none of the earlier descriptive postmortem studies noted neuronal loss. This apparent absence of neuronal loss has led to the recent undertaking of quantitative microscopic studies of the brain. Such studies are not only complex and time consuming but are prone to a number of confounding technical problems[81,82]. These include: 1) the influence of shrinkage and age – both of these can cause considerable volume changes during both fixation and embedding of tissue blocks in paraffin wax. The degree of shrinkage is idiosyncratic to the individual, age dependent, and influenced by the chemicals used during the preparation. The importance of shrinkage is that it can substantially alter the apparent number of neurons; 2) tissue section thickness can produce optical distortions that affect cell number and size, the thicker the section the worse the distortions; 3) the complex structure and organization of neurons within the brain, called anisotropy, mean that obtaining a representative sample requires complicated techniques.

Ketzler et al.[83] examined the frontal cortex of 18 patients who had died of AIDS, using computer assisted image analysis. The neuronal density was found to be reduced by 18% in the AIDS brains compared to controls. However, the study was indiscriminate as the brains were examined regardless of the neuropathological diagnoses, thus it was not possible to state whether the neuronal loss resulted from HIV infection or coincidental, and often multiple, pathology. The issue was clarified in a study which excluded cases with opportunistic infections or neoplasms. The study examined the frontal cortex from 11 HIV infected cases (5 cases with a neuropathological diagnosis of HIV encephalitis and 6 with only minimal pathology) and compared these to 8 age–sex matched controls[68]. Employing a stereological technique called the 'disector'[84], apt for brain quantitation, the study revealed a loss of 38% in the density of neurons in the frontal cortex in HIV infected brains. This result was confirmed when the study was repeated using computer assisted image analysis; this method found a loss of approximately 35%[85].

This study showed neuronal loss most likely caused by HIV. Secondly, the neuronal loss occurred regardless of whether there was encephalitis or only minimal pathology, hence indicating that the neuronal loss and the inflammation may be two independent processes. These findings were confirmed by an independent method. Recently, a computer assisted image analysis study of different cortical areas (frontal, temporal and parietal) found a 30–50% loss of neurons depending on size and brain region[86].

Mechanisms of neuronal loss

The recognition of substantial neuronal loss requires explanation of pathogenesis as there is no evidence for neuronal infection by HIV[39]. In addition, if the mechanism of neuronal loss were reversible, HIV dementia could be treated or even prevented. Currently, all work on neurotoxicity has been carried out in cell culture. There are a number of proposed etiologies of neurotoxicity. They are outlined as follows:

Cofactors The presence of opportunistic infections could act as a cofactor in promoting severe encephalitis. Systemically, coinfection with other infectious agents can enhance HIV expression by a mechanism similar to that seen with *tat*, the HIV gene regulating viral expression[18]. Gene expression can be stimulated by simultaneous infection of HIV infected cells by cytomegalovirus, herpes simplex virus types 1 and 2, human herpes virus type 6, and Epstein–Barr virus[21]. Both JC virus[24] and the human herpes virus-6[23] have been demonstrated to have a cofactor role in the brain.

Cytokines An excess production of cytokines may result in brain tissue damage. One such cytokine is α-tumour necrosis factor (α-TNF), which is elevated in the spinal fluid in HIV infected patients. Astrocytes can be activated to produce α-TNF[87], and this production can, in turn, increase the expression of HIV[88]. In addition, this factor damages oligodendrocytes in culture and disrupts myelin; these changes may progress to demyelination[89]. The involvement of other cytokines is supported by the observation that HIV infected macrophages, which are the main reservoir of HIV in the brain, produce a soluble factor, called contrainterleukin-1 which blocks interleukin-1 mediated T cell activation[90]. HIV infected macrophages produce other soluble factors[91] and macrophages can cause secretion of immune mediators including cytokines, prostaglandins, leukotrienes, kyneurines, oxidative radicals and proteases. All of these immune mediators have the potential for deleterious effects on cellular functioning.

Alterations in brain metabolism A number of abnormalities have been detected. Examination of cerebrospinal fluid has revealed lower concentrations of S-adenosylmethionine (SAM) and raised levels of S-adenosylhomocysteine (SAH), and therefore a lower methylation ratio SAM/SAH, in HIV infected patients[92]. A reduced methylation ratio inhibits brain methyltransferase as this enzyme is highly dependent on the concentration of the methyl donor SAM and inhibited by high concentrations of the product of the methylation reaction, SAH. This enzyme system is also dependent on vitamin B12 and there is some similarity between the demyelinating lesions seen in B12 deficiency and those induced by HIV. It is therefore thought that the disturbance in methyltransferase enzymes observed in HIV infection could result in hypomethylation of myelin and thence demyelination, which, in turn, manifests as neurological disturbance. In addition, the ^{31}P MRS study discussed earlier found that HIV infected individuals had a lower adenosine triphosphate to inorganic phosphate ratio[57], and this was due to impaired brain cellular oxidative metabolism. There also appeared to be a correlation between the depressed ratio and the severity of the dementia. However, it is still not clear whether this metabolic alteration is specific to HIV disease or whether it occurs in other diseases.

Nonspecific mechanisms There may be nonspecific, or poorly characterized, events that either directly injure neurons, such as toxic factors, or may damage glial cells, resulting in secondary changes such as impaired metabolism or demyelination. One nonspecific finding is an increase in laminin in capillary walls in the HIV infected brain[93]. It is thought that, as HIV may enter the brain through the capillaries, laminin occurs in response to damage to the capillary and may indicate disruption of the blood–brain barrier which, in turn, may result in impaired neuronal function.

HIV gene products These may interfere with neuronal function. The toxicity of viral products is also indicated by the report of high levels of unintegrated HIV viral DNA in brain tissue with HIV encephalitis[94]. Retroviral DNA can exist in host cells in three forms: unintegrated linear, unintegrated circular, and integrated. High levels of the unintegrated form often correlate with superinfection and cytopathicity[95].

HIV envelope glycoprotein gp120 This has been reported to inhibit the function of neuroleukin, a growth factor required for neuronal survival[96]. Gp120 may also have neurotoxic action as it kills fetal rodent hippocampal neurons in culture[97]. However, it is not known whether gp120 acts directly on neurons or whether the toxicity is mediated by binding to glial cells and inducing production of toxins. It is reported that gp120 causes, in rats, a global reduction in cerebral glucose utilization[98] which is reminiscent of the findings in patients with AIDS dementia complex, by positron emission tomography[99].

The neurotoxic effect of gp120 can be blocked by gp120 antibodies but not by anti-CD4 antibodies[100], and it is unlikely that neurons have CD4 receptors. The neuronal damage can be prevented by 2 neurotransmitters: vasoactive intestinal peptide (VIP) and peptide T[97]. Gp120 shares sequence homology with both VIP and Peptide T and it is thought that gp120 competes with VIP for VIPergic neuronal receptors. Gp120 fragments themselves might be active as indicated by the finding that not even proteases alter the toxic effect of the secreted macrophage toxic factor/s[101].

The hypothesis that gp120 or a gp120 fragment may induce neurotoxicity by attachment to a VIP receptor is too simplistic. It is known that VIP causes oscillations in the entry of calcium into neurons and that attachment of gp120 causes a rise in intracellular calcium followed, after a delay, by cell death. The large rise in intracellular calcium is postulated to trigger a lethal set of events[102], including lipid peroxidation, free radical formation, degradation of cytoskeletal proteins, and DNA fragmentation. The gp120 induced calcium entry can be blocked by calcium channel antagonists, ie nifedipine and nimopidine[103], and by antagonists of the N-methyl-D-aspartate (NMDA) receptor, which is a subtype of the glutamate receptor[102]. The glutamate receptor population consists of subtypes: NMDA and non-NMDA receptors. While antagonists to NMDA receptors effectively block the gp120 induced toxicity, antagonists to non-NMDA receptors are ineffective. These findings indicate that the toxicity appears to be dependent on calcium entry through 2 different calcium channels: a voltage dependent channel that can be blocked by calcium antagonists, and a calcium channel coupled to the NMDA receptor. Activation of the NMDA calcium channel and the presence of gp120 both seem essential to induce neurotoxicity. If exogenous glutamate is added in high concentrations to cultured neuronal cells, there is no toxicity. However, if gp120 is added to the cultured cells, together with glutamate, there is neuronal death. This death can be prevented by first degrading the endogenous glutamate in the cell culture; in this circumstance gp120 does not induce any toxicity[104]. Thus gp120 and glutamate are synergistic neurotoxins. In vivo there is an endogenous NMDA agonist, quinolinic acid. Quinolinic acid has been found to be elevated in the CSF of patients with HIV infection, and there was some evidence that the concentrations of quinolinic acid paralleled the severity of the cognitive and motor dysfunction[105]. Therefore elevated quinolinic acid may act as an excitotoxin activating the NMDA receptor which, in HIV infected individuals, has a synergistic action with gp120 and thus mediates neuronal injury and death.

Conclusions

It is now well established that HIV causes significant damage to the brain, as indicated by neuropathology, neuroimaging and neuropsychology. Clinically, there is a severe dementia that is only now being clarified and defined more rigorously. This clarification should also include joint clinical and neuropathological agreement on the concept of HIV associated dementia being considered a subcortical dementia. Even though early postmortem studies[78] supported the notion that the HIV induced lesions are limited to the subcortical areas further studies, including those demonstrating cortical neuronal loss, do not support this view.

Current research needs to be addressed to four main areas. First, definitive clinical and neuropathological entities of HIV induced disease need to be agreed. Secondly, a secure nomenclature in the two areas will then facilitate investigation of how these different abnormalities correlate with one another and which neuropsychological, neuroimaging, or neuropathological abnormalities are clinically significant and result in dysfunction. Thirdly, such correlations will further understanding of the cause of the HIV associated dementia. Lastly, examination of the cellular and molecular mechanisms which may underlie neuronal loss and hence the dementia is required. Essentially there are four theories: the virus can act directly on neurons, or it can act via astrocytes, or via macrophages and microglia, or there may be a combination of the above three. It seems that the toxicity is dependent on gp120 and NMDA receptor activation, however, the role of VIP, peptide T, cytokines and other factors remains to be elucidated. Understanding of each cellular mechanism may provide therapeutic avenues for prevention or even reversal of the neuronal loss and cognitive dysfunction.

References

(1) Center for Disease Control. Pneumocystis pneumonia. *Los Angeles, Morbidity Mortality Weekly Rep* 1981; 30 (Jun 5): 250–2.
(2) Center for Disease Control. Kaposi's sarcoma and pneumocystis pneumonia among homosexual men. *NY City California, Morbidity Mortality Weekly Rep* 1981; 30 (Jul 3): 305–8.
(3) Snider WD, Simpson DM, Nielsen S, Gold JWM, Metroka CE, Posner JB. Neurological complications of acquired immune deficiency syndrome: analysis of 50 patients. *Ann Neurol* 1983; 14: 403–18.
(4) Barre-Sinoussi F, Chermann JC, Rey F et al. Isolation of a T-lymphotropic retrovirus from a patient at risk for acquired immune deficiency syndrome (AIDS). *Science* 1983; 220: 868–71.
(5) Gallo RC, Sarin PS, Gelmann EP et al. Isolation of human T-cell leukaemia virus in acquired immune deficiency syndrome (AIDS). *Science* 1983; 220: 865–7.
(6) Maj M. Organic mental disorders in HIV-1 infection. *AIDS* 1990; 4: 831–40.
(7) Everall IP, Lantos PL. The neuropathology of HIV. *Int Rev Psychiat* 1991; 3: 307–20.
(8) Dalgleish A, Beverley P, Clapham , Crawford DH, Greaves MF, Weiss RW. The CD4 (T4) antigen is an essential component of the receptor for the AIDS retrovirus. *Nature* 1984; 312: 763–6.
(9) Klatzmann D, Champagne E, Chamaret S et al. T-lymphocyte T4 molecule behaves as a receptor for human retrovirus LAV. *Nature* 1984; 312: 767–71.
(10) Klatzmann D, Barre-Sinoussi F, Nugeyre MT et al. Selective tropism of lymphadenopathy-associated virus (LAV) for helper-inducer T lymphocytes. *Science* 1984; 225: 59–62.
(11) Levy JA, Shimabukuro J, McHugh T, Casavant C, Stites D, Oshiro L. AIDS-associated retroviruses (ARV) can productively infect other cells besides human T-helper cells. *Virology* 1985; 147: 441–8.
(12) Homsy J, Meyer M, Tateno M, Clarkson S, Levy JA. The Fc and not the CD4 receptor mediates antibody enhancement of HIV infection in human cells. *Science* 1989; 244: 1357–60.
(13) Robinson WE, Montefiori DC, Mitchell WM. Antibody dependent enhancement of human immunodeficiency virus type-1 infection. *Lancet* 1988; i: 790–5.
(14) Rosen CA, Sodroski JG, Goh WC, Dayton AI, Lippke J, Hasletine WA. Posttranscriptional regulation accounts for the trans-activation of the human T-lymphotropic virus type III. *Nature* 1986; 319: 555–9.

(15) O'Brien WA, Koyanagi Y, Chen ISY. Virologic aspects of AIDS and the nervous system. In: Vinters HV, Anders KH, eds. *Neuropathology of AIDS*. Florida: CRC Press, 1990: 189–207.

(16) Levy JA. Changing concepts in HIV infection: challenges for the 1990s. *AIDS* 1990; 4: 1051–8.

(17) Strebel K, Daugherty D, Clouse K, Cohen D, Folks T, Martin MA. The HIV 'A' (sor) gene product is essential for virus infectivity. *Nature* 1987; 328: 728–00.

(18) O'Brien WA, Zack JA, Chen ISY. Molecular pathogenesis of HIV-1. *AIDS* 1990; 4(Suppl): S41–8.

(19) Jones KA, Kadonaga JT, Luciw PA, Tijan R. Activation of the AIDS retrovirus promotor by the cellular transcription factor, Spl. *Science* 1986; 232: 755–9.

(20) Garcia JA, Wu FK, Mitsuyasu RT, Gaynor RB. Interactions of cellular proteins involved in the transcriptional regulation of human immunodeficiency virus. *EMBO J* 1987; 6: 3761–70.

(21) Laurence J. Molecular interactions among herpes viruses and human immunodeficiency viruses. *J Infec Dis* 1990; 162: 338–46.

(22) Montagnier L. HIV pathogenesis. *VI International Conference on AIDS, Final Program and Abstracts*, vol. 1, San Francisco, USA, 1990: 150.

(23) Lusso P, Ensoli B, Markham PD et al. Productive dual infection of human CD4+ T lymphocytes by HIV-1 and HHV-6. *Nature* 1989; 337: 370–3.

(24) Vazeux R, Cumont M, Girard PM et al. Severe encephalitis resulting from coinfections with HIV and JC virus. *Neurology* 1990; 40: 944–8.

(25) Alizon M, Wain-Hobson S, Montagnier L, Sonigo P. Genetic variability of the AIDS virus: nucleotide sequence analysis of two isolates from African patients. *Cell* 1986; 46: 63–74.

(26) Hahn BH, Shaw GM, Taylor ME et al. Genetic variation in HTLV-III/LAV over time in patients with AIDS or at risk from AIDS. *Science* 1986; 232: 1548–53.

(27) Starcich BR, Hahn BH, Shaw GM et al. Identification and characterization of conserved and variable regions in the envelope gene of HTLV-III/LAV, the retrovirus of AIDS. *Cell* 1986; 45: 637–48.

(28) Gartner S, Markovitz P, Markovitz DM. The role of mononuclear phagocytes in HTLV III/LAV infection. *Science* 1986; 234: 1563–6.

(29) Cheng-Mayer C, Levy JA. Distinct biological and serological properties of human immunodeficiency viruses from the brain. *Ann Neurol* 1988; 23: S58–61.

(30) Cordonnier A, Montagnier L, Emerman M. Single amino-acid changes in HIV envelope affect viral tropism and receptor binding. *Nature* 1989; 340: 571–4.

(31) Meltzler MS, Nakamura M, Hansen BD, Turpin JA, Kalter DC, Gendelman HE. Macrophages as susceptible targets for HIV infection, persistent viral reservoirs in tissue and key immunoregulatory cells that control levels of virus replication and extent of disease. *AIDS Res Hum Retroviruses* 1990; 6: 967–71.

(32) Ho DD, Rota TR, Schooley RT et al. Isolation of HTLV-III from cerebrospinal fluid and neural tissues of patients with neurologic syndromes related to the acquired immunodeficiency syndrome. *N Eng J Med* 1985; 313: 1493–7.

(33) Peluso R, Haase A, Stowring L, Edwards M, Ventura P. A Trojan horse mechanism for the spread of visna virus in monocytes. *Virology* 1985; 147: 231–6.

(34) Wiley CA, Schrier RD, Nelson JA, Lampert PW, Oldstone MBA. Cellular localisation of human immunodeficiency virus infection within the brains of acquired immune deficiency syndrome patients. *Proc Nat Acad Sci USA* 1986; 83: 7089–93.

(35) Harouse JM, Wroblewska Z, Laughlin MA, Schonwetter BS, Gonzalez-Scarano F. Human choroid plexus cells can be latently infected with human immunodeficiency virus. *Ann Neurol* 1989; 4: 406–11.

(36) Epstein LG, Sharer LR, Cho ES, Meyenhofer MF, Navia BA, Price RW. HTLV III/LAV-like retrovirus particles in the brains of patients with AIDS encephalopathy. *AIDS Res* 1985; 1: 447–54.

(37) Pumarola-Sune T, Navia BA, Cordon-Cardo C, Cho ES, Price RW. HIV antigen in the brains of patients with the AIDS dementia complex. *Ann Neurol* 1987; 21: 490–6.

(38) Stoler MH, Eskin TA, Benn S, Angerer RC, Angerer LM. Human T-cell lymphotropic virus type III infection of the central nervous system. A preliminary in situ analysis. *J Am Med Assn* 1986; 256: 2381–3.

(39) Michaels J, Sharer LR, Epstein LG. Human immunodeficiency virus type 1 (HIV-1) infection of the nervous system: a review. *Immunodefic Rev* 1988; 1: 71–104.

(40) Catalan J. Psychiatric manifestations of HIV disease. *Baillière's Clin Gastroenterol* 1990; 4: 547–62.

(41) Navia BA, Jordan BD, Price RW. The AIDS dementia complex I: clinical features. *Ann Neurol* 1986; 19: 517–24.

(42) Price RW, Sidtis JJ, Brew B. AIDS dementia complex and HIV-1 infection: a view from the clinic. *Brain Pathol* 1991; 1: 155–62.

(43) American Academy of Neurology AIDS Task Force. Nomenclature and research case definitions for neurologic manifestations of human immunodeficiency virus-type 1 (HIV-1) infection. *Neurology* 1991; 41: 778–85.

(44) Belman AL, Ultmann MH, Horoupian D et al. Neurological complications in infants and children with acquired immune deficiency syndrome. *Ann Neurol* 1985; 18: 560–6.

(45) Tross S, Price RW, Navia B et al. Neuropsychological characterization of the AIDS dementia complex: a preliminary report. *AIDS* 1988; 2: 81–8.

(46) Grant I, Atkinson JH, Hesselink JR et al. Evidence for early central nervous system involvement in the acquired immunodeficiency syndrome (AIDS) and other human immunodeficiency virus (HIV) infections. Studies with neuropsychologic testing and magnetic resonance imaging. *Ann Intern Med* 1987; 107: 828–36.

(47) Harter DH. Neuropsychological status of asymptomatic individuals seropositive to HIV-1. *Ann Neurol* 1989; 26: 589–91.

(48) Saykin AJ, Janssen RS, Sprehn GC, Gwen C, Kaplan JE. Neuropsychological dysfunction in HIV infection: characterization in a lymphadenopathy cohort. *Int J Clin Neuropsychol* 1988; 10: 81–95.

I P Everall and P L Lantos

(49) Janssen RS, Saykin AJ, Cannon L et al. Neurological and neuropsychological manifestations of HIV-1 infection: association with AIDS-related complex but not asymptomatic HIV-1 infection. *Ann Neurol* 1989; 26: 592–600.
(50) McArthur JC, Cohen BA, Selnes OA et al. Low prevalence of neurological and neuropsychological abnormalities in otherwise healthy HIV-1 infected individuals: results from the multicenter AIDS cohort study. *Ann Neurol* 1989; 26: 601–11.
(51) Catalan J. HIV-associated dementia. *Int Rev Psychiat* 1991; 3: 321–30.
(52) Chrysikopoulos H, Press G, Grafe M, Hesselink J, Wiley C. Encephalitis caused by HIV: CT and MRI manifestations with clinical and pathological correlation. *Neuroradiology* 1990; 175: 185–91.
(53) Vinters HV, Anders KH. Introduction and overview. In: Vinters HV, Anders KH, eds. *Neuropathology of AIDS*. Florida: CRC Press, 1990: 1–20.
(54) Post J, Tate L, Quencer R et al. CT, MR, and pathology in HIV encephalitis and meningitis. *Am J Radiol* 1988; 151: 373–80.
(55) Singer E, Syndulko K, Ruane P et al. Magnetic resonance imaging findings in human immunodeficiency virus-positive and high risk seronegative individuals. *Ann Neurol* 1989; 26: 154–5.
(56) Sonnerberg A, Saaf J, Alexius B, Strannegard O, Wahlund LO, Wetterberg L. Quantitative detection of brain aberrations in human immunodeficiency virus type 1 infected individuals by magnetic resonance imaging. *J Infec Dis* 1990; 162: 1245–51.
(57) Deicken RF, Hubesch B, Jensen PC et al. Alterations in brain phosphate metabolite concentrations in patients with human immunodeficiency virus infection. *Arch Neurol* 1991; 48: 203–9.
(58) Menon DK, Baudouin CJ, Tomlinson D, Hoyle C. Proton spectroscopy and imaging of the brain in AIDS: evidence of neuronal loss in regions that appear normal with imaging. *J Comp Assisted Tomog* 1990; 14: 882–5.
(59) Nadler JV, Cooper JR. N-acetyl-L-aspartic acid content of human neural tumours bovine peripheral nervous tissues. *J Neurochem* 1972; 19: 313–19.
(60) Maini CL, Pigorini F, Pau FM et al. Cortical cerebral blood flow in HIV-1 related dementia complex. 1990; 11: 639–48.
(61) Kuni CC, Rhame FS, Meier MJ et al. Quantitative I-123-IMP brain SPECT and neuropsychological testing in AIDS dementia. *Clin Nucl Med* 1991; 16: 174–7.
(62) Kramer EL, Sanger JJ. Brain imaging in acquired immunodeficiency syndrome dementia complex. *Sem Nucl Med* 1990; 20: 353–63.
(63) Tatsch K, Schielke E, Bauer WM, Markl A, Einhaupl KM, Kirsch CM. Functional and morphological findings in early and advanced stages of HIV infection: a comparison of 99mTc-HMPAO SPECT with CT and MRI studies. *Nuklearmedizin* 1990; 29: 252–8.
(64) Budka H, Wiley CA, Kleihues P et al. HIV-associated disease of the nervous system and proposal for neuropathology-based terminology. *Brain Pathol* 1991; 1: 143–52.
(65) Shaw GM, Harper ME, Hahn BH et al. HTLV-III infection in the brains of children and adults with AIDS encephalopathy. *Science* 1985; 227: 177–82.

(66) Budka H. Neuropathology of human immunodeficiency virus infection. *Brain Pathol* 1991; 1: 163–75.

(67) Budka H, Costanzi G, Cristina S et al. Brain pathology induced by infection with human immunodeficiency virus (HIV). A histological, immunocytochemical, and electron microscopical study of 100 autopsy cases. *Acta Neuropathol* 1987; 75: 185–98.

(68) Everall IP, Luthert PJ, Lantos PL. Neuronal loss in the frontal cortex in HIV infection. *Lancet* 1991; 337: 1119–21.

(69) Kleihues P, Lang W, Burger PC et al. Progressive diffuse leukoencephalopathy in patients with acquired immune deficiency syndrome. *J Neuropathol Exp Neurol* 1985; 50: 171–83.

(70) Kaus J, Zurlinden B, Schlote W. Axonal volume and myelin sheath thickness of central nervous system myelinated fibres are reduced in HIV-encephalopathy. *Clin Neuropathol* 1991; 10: 38.

(71) Smith TW, DeGirolami U, Henin D, Bolgert F, Hauw J-J. Human immunodeficiency virus (HIV) leukoencephalopathy and the microcirculation. *J Neuropathol Exp Neurol* 1990; 49: 357–70.

(72) Petito CK, Navia BA, Cho ES, Jordan BD, George DC, Price RW. Vacuolar myelopathy pathologically resembling subacute combined degeneration in patients with the acquired immunodeficiency syndrome. *N Eng J Med* 1985; 312: 874–9.

(73) Budka H. Human immunodeficiency virus (HIV)-induced disease of the central nervous system: pathology and implications for pathogenesis. *Acta Neuropathol* 1990; 77: 225–36.

(74) Lenhardt TM, Super MA, Wiley CA. Neuropathological changes in an asymptomatic HIV seropositive man. *Ann Neurol* 1988; 23: 209–10.

(75) Esiri MM, Scaravilli F, Millard PR, Harcourt-Webster JN. Neuropathology of HIV infection in haemophiliacs: comparative necropsy study. *Br Med J* 1990; 299: 1312–15.

(76) Lantos PL, McLaughlin JE, Scholtz CL, Berry CL, Tighe JR. Neuropathology of the brain in HIV infection. *Lancet* 1989; i: 309–11.

(77) Gray F, Gherardi R, Lescs MC et al. Early brain changes in HIV infection: neuropathologic study of 11 HIV-seropositive, non-AIDS asymptomatic cases, neuroscience of HIV infection basic and clinical frontiers. *Satellite Conference the seventh international conference on AIDS*. Padova, Italy, 1991: 35.

(78) Navia BA, Cho ES, Petito CK, Price RW. The AIDS dementia complex II. Neuropathology. *Ann Neurol* 1986; 19: 525–35.

(79) Price RW, Brew B, Sidtis J, Rosenblum M, Scheck AC, Cleary P. The brain in AIDS: central nervous system HIV-1 infection and AIDS dementia complex. *Science* 1988; 239: 586–92.

(80) Moeller AA, Backmund HC. Ventricle and brain ratio in the clinical course of HIV infection. *Acta Neurol Scand* 1990; 81: 512–15.

(81) Aherne WA, Dunnill MS. *Morphometry*. London: Edward Arnold, 1982.

(82) Haug H. History of neuromorphometry. *J Neurosci Meth* 1986; 18: 1–17.

(83) Ketzler S, Weis S, Haug H, Budka H. Loss of neurons in the frontal cortex in AIDS brains. *Acta Neuropathol* 1990; 80: 92–4.

(84) Sterio DC. The unbiased estimation of number and sizes of arbitrary particles using the disector. *J Microscopy* 1984; 134: 127–36.

(85) Everall IP, Luthert PJ, Lantos PL. Cell population changes in the putamen and frontal cortex in HIV infection. *Neuropathol Appl Neurobiol* 1991; 17: 246.

(86) Wiley CA, Masliah E, Morey M et al. Neocortical damage during HIV infection. *Ann Neurol* 1991; 29: 651–7.

(87) Grimaldi LME, Martino GV, Franciotta DM et al. Elevated alpha-tumor necrosis factor levels in spinal fluid from HIV-1 infected patients with central nervous system involvement. *Ann Neurol* 1991; 29: 21–5.

(88) Osborn L, Kunkel S, Nabel GJ. Tumour necrosis factor α and interleukin 1 stimulate the human immunodeficiency enhancer by activation of nuclear factor kB. *Proc Nat Acad Sci USA* 1989; 86: 2336–40.

(89) Selmaj KW, Raine CS. Tumour necrosis factor mediates myelin and oligodendrocytes damage in vitro. *Ann Neurol* 1988; 23: 339–46.

(90) Locksley RM, Crowe S, Saddick MD et al. Release of interleukin I inhibitory activity (contra IL-1) by human monocyte derived macrophages infected with human immunodeficiency virus in vitro and in vivo. *J Clin Invest* 1988; 82: 2097–105.

(91) Pulliam L, Herndier BG, Tang NM, McGrath MS. Human immunodeficiency virus-infected macrophages produce soluble factors that cause histological and neurochemical alterations in cultured human brains. *J Clin Invest* 1991; 87: 503–12.

(92) Keating JN, Trimble KC, Mulchay F, Scott JM, Weir DG. Evidence of brain methyltransferase inhibition and early brain involvement in HIV-positive patients. *Lancet* 1991; 337: 935–9.

(93) Taruscio D, Malchiodi Abedi F, Bagnato R et al. Increased reactivity of laminin in the basement membranes of capillary walls in AIDS brain cortex. *Acta Neuropathol* 1991; 81: 552–6.

(94) Pang S, Koyanagi Y, Miles S, Wiley C, Vinters H, Chen ISY. High levels of unintegrated HIV-1 DNA in brain tissue of AIDS dementia patients. *Nature* 1990; 343: 85–9.

(95) Mullins JI, Chen CS, Hoover EA. Disease-specific and tissue-specific production of unintegrated feline leukaemia virus variant DNA in feline AIDS. *Nature* 1986; 319: 333–6.

(96) Wahl LM, Corcoran ML, Pyle SW, Arthur LO, Harel-Bellan A, Farrar WL. Human immunodeficiency virus glycoprotein (gp120) induction of monocyte arachidonic acid metabolites and interleukin 1. *Proc Nat Acad Sci USA* 1989; 86: 621–5.

(97) Brenneman DE, Westbrook GL, Fitzgerald SP et al. Neuronal cell killing by the envelope protein and its prevention by vasoactive peptide. *Nature* 1988; 335: 639–42.

(98) Kimes AS, London ED, Szabo G, Raymon L, Tabakoff B. Reduction of cerebral glucose utilisation by the HIV envelope glycoprotein gp120. *Exp Neurol* 1991; 112: 224–8.

(99) Rottenberg DA, Moeller JR, Strother SC et al. The metabolic pathology of the AIDS dementia complex. *Ann Neurol* 1987; 22: 700–6.

(100) Kaiser PK, Offermann JT, Lipton SA. Neuronal injury due to HIV-1 is

blocked by anti-gp120 antibodies but not by anti-CD4 antibodies. *Neurology* 1990; 40: 1757–61.

(101) Giulian D, Vaca K, Noonan CA. Secretion of neurotoxins by mononuclear phagocytes infected with HIV-1. *Science* 1990; 250: 1593–6.

(102) Lipton SA. HIV-related neurotoxicity. *Brain Pathol* 1991; 1: 193–9.

(103) Dreyer EB, Kaiser PK, Offermann JT, Lipton SA. HIV-1 coat protein neurotoxicity prevented by calcium channel antagonists. *Science* 1990; 248: 364–7.

(104) Lipton SA, Sucher NJ, Kaiser PK, Dreyer EB. Synergistic effects of HIV coat protein and NMDA receptor-mediated neurotoxicity. *Neuron* 1991; 7: 111–18.

(105) Heyes MP, Brew BJ, Martin A et al. Quinolinic acid in cerebrospinal fluid and serum in HIV-1 infection: relationship to clinical and neurological status. *Ann Neurol* 1991; 29: 202–9.

Magnetic resonance spectroscopy: applications in psychiatry

M S KESHAVAN and J W PETTEGREW

It has been stated that one of the major roadblocks to progress in understanding of the cerebral basis of mental disorders is the human skull[1]! Until recently, direct access to the human brain for research studies was mainly via postmortem studies. The application of brain imaging techniques such as computerized tomography and magnetic resonance imaging (MRI) have transformed the scene in psychiatric research. The advent of 'physiological' or 'functional' techniques such as positron emission tomography (PET) and magnetic resonance spectroscopy (MRS), is relatively recent. MRS is a noninvasive in vivo approach to measure important metabolites in living tissues, and is based on the principle of nuclear magnetic resonance (NMR). MRS has great potential for the study of the molecular dynamics and metabolic state both in vitro and in vivo. In this chapter, we have reviewed the history and basic physical principles of magnetic resonance, the techniques, and the chemical insights provided by MRS as well as its potential applications to psychiatry. We will focus on currently published in vivo MRS studies of psychiatric disorders. For more exhaustive reviews of this rapidly expanding field, the interested reader is referred to more elaborate texts[1-11].

Historical background

Purcell and Bloch[12,13] working independently, were the first to discover that the magnetic dipoles of molecules in matter resonate in response to an externally applied field (nuclear magnetic resonance, or NMR). Bloch also observed that nuclei resonating to an external magnetic field induce an electromotive force in a surrounding recording coil. The Nobel prize for physics was awarded to Bloch and Purcell in 1952 for these pioneering observations[14]. Biological applications began soon thereafter; Bloch demonstrated a strong NMR signal from his finger inserted into the radio frequency (RF) coil of his

All correspondence to: Dr M S Keshavan, University of Pittsburgh, Department of Psychiatry, Western Psychiatric Institute and Clinic, 3811 O'Hara Street, Pittsburgh, PA 15213, USA

Cambridge Medical Reviews: Neurobiology and Psychiatry Volume 2
© Cambridge University Press

spectrometer. In 1948, Purcell recorded signals generated by his own dental fillings. Other advances in biological application of MRS had to await the development of strong field, high resolution magnets, Fourier transformation software, as well as the introduction of surface coil technology. Moon and Richards (1974) conducted ^{31}P MRS studies of erythrocytes[15]. Hoult et al. obtained a ^{31}P MRS from rat leg muscle[16]. Human limbs were then studied, enabled by the advent of superconducting magnets; infant head was studied before the technique was used to study adult brains because of magnet bore size limitations[17.]

MRS has seemed to have lagged behind MRI[18], perhaps due to more stringent technical requirements. Another possible reason is that in contrast to MRI where the anatomical database is well known, data on diverse biochemical information needed to interpret MRS findings is sorely lacking. In vitro MRS has long been studied as a tool for analytical chemistry in research laboratories that have high resolution magnets which may not have the capacity for human in vivo studies. The use of in vivo MRS in clinical settings has blossomed largely over the last decade.

What is nuclear magnetic resonance?

Atoms contain nuclei that comprise different numbers of protons and neutrons. All nuclei which have either an odd number of protons or neutrons have a spin, in a way similar to the earth's spin around its axis. [1]H has a core of only one proton, and [7]Li has 3 protons and 4 neutrons. These nuclei spin about an axis generating a small magnetic field (Fig. 1). Each nucleus with a charge and a spin can be likened to a small bar magnet. However, not every atom has a spin, eg ^{1}H with one proton has a spin but in [4]He 2 protons and 2 neutrons cancel each other's spin. Only atoms with net spins, eg ^{1}H, ^{13}C, ^{19}F, [23]Na, ^{31}P lend themselves to NMR studies.

In the absence of an external magnetic field, all atoms in matter are randomly aligned. When placed in an external magnetic field (B_0), the tiny magnets line up along the direction of the magnetic field like a compass needle in the earth's magnetic field (Fig. 2). In this state matter can be considered to be made up of multiple tops, all spinning about the axis of the

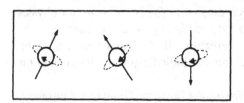

Fig. 1. Matter as shown here is composed of multiple nucleons. These are charged and have a net spin, (spin shown by dotted arrows), they act like tiny magnetic dipoles, (represented by slid arrow). At rest, all dipoles are arranged randomly.

196

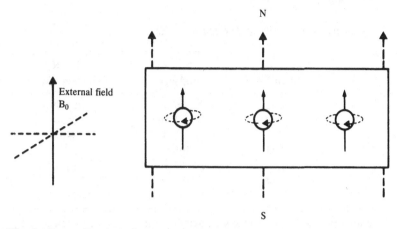

Fig. 2. On application of an external field, B_0, the magnetic dipoles (solid arrow), arrange themselves along the direction of the external field (broken arrow).

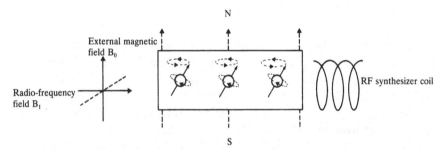

Fig. 3. On application of an additional radio frequency field, B_1, the dipoles already aligned along B_0 now start 'precessing' around axis B_0.

external field (z axis). If another field B_1, generated by a RF coil is now applied, at an angle of 90° to B_0, the spinning tops can be 'tipped' in the x–y axis, thus being elevated to a higher state of energy; the nuclei which were initially spinning around the B_0 axis will start 'precessing' around that axis in addition, like a top spinning about the spike (Fig. 3).

In a given magnetic field, each distinct nuclear species resonates at a unique frequency, the Larmor frequency. This frequency varies with the external magnetic field as well as the properties of the nucleus. Thus, it is derived by the equation $W = \dfrac{\gamma B_0}{2\pi}$, where

W = resonating frequency (frequency of applied RF field)
γ = gyromagnetic constant
B_0 = externally applied static field.

M S Keshavan and J W Pettegrew

Table 1. *List of nuclei that can be detected by MRS*

Element	Intrinsic sensitivity (%)	Natural abundance (%)	NMR frequency (MHz)
^{1}H	100.00	99.885	100.00
^{13}C	1.59	1.108	25.14
^{19}F	83.4	100.00	94.09
^{23}Na	9.24	100.00	26.45
^{39}K	5.08	93.1	4.67
^{31}P	6.64	100.00	40.48
^{7}Li	27	92.58	38.86

'Intrinsic sensitivity' reveals the relative sensitivity of a given isotope to detection by MRS. 'Natural abundance' expresses in percentage the extent to which the listed isotope constitutes the element as present in the human body under natural conditions.

The strength of the earth's magnetic field is approximately half a gauss; 10 000 gauss equals 1 tesla. In an external magnetic field of 2.35 tesla, the resonating frequency for ^{1}H is 100.00 MHz and that for ^{31}P is 40.48 MHz (Table 1). Thus, in a chemical mixture which contains ^{1}H and ^{31}P, one can selectively apply a radio frequency of 100.00 MHz, and resonate only ^{1}H, or apply a radio frequency of 40.48 MHz and resonate only ^{31}P.

If RF field is now removed, the nuclei return to their original axis ('relaxation') (Fig. 4). This change of orientation of these tops, in the presence of the external magnetic field B_0 induces a voltage signal in a recording coil around this material; the signal recorded varies with time as it decays. This phenomenon is called free induction decay (or the FID). By a mathematical process called Fourier transformation, one can extract frequency information from FID. (This is similar to prism breaking light into the various colour components.) T_1 and T_2, relaxation times, are sample related measures of the rate of decay of this signal. The component of the relaxation to the z axis is termed longitudinal or spin–lattice relaxation, or T_1, and the relaxation in the $(x-y)$ axis is termed spin–spin relaxation, or T_2. It is of significance that the relaxation times in body water are altered in pathological states. By generating MR images where intensity of signal depends on the relaxation times, one can obtain valuable information about brain pathology.

NMR principles as applied to MRI

MRI depends on the principle that the Larmor frequency varies with the strength of the external magnetic field. If the field varies over a gradient in the sample being studied, the NMR signal from a given nucleus will depend on

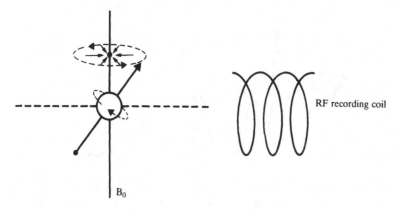

Fig. 4. On removal of the radio frequency field, the 'precessing' dipole returns to alignment along axis B_0. This process called relaxation, is characterized by T_1 and T_2 (see text) and induces an electromotive force in the recording coil.

its spatial position in the sample. It is possible to create a picture of the proton concentration in the sample by appropriate manipulation of the B_0 field. By altering parameters associated with data generation, images emphasizing either T_1 or T_2 relaxation times, can be obtained; such images provide valuable information about different types of tissue pathology. This is the basis of MRI.

NMR principles as applied to MRS

A different principle is exploited by MRS. The resonance frequency of a nucleus is also affected by the local magnetic field of the molecular 'cloud' of electrons surrounding the nucleus; this effect is called the chemical shift, and is described in units of parts per million (ppm), ie millionths of the Larmor frequency in relation to a central radio frequency. Thus, the same element in different chemical compounds resonates at slightly different frequencies. By using Fourier transformation, the resultant FID can be analysed for the frequencies contained in it, in order to produce a spectrum. The spectrum provides information as to what biochemicals are present by the position of the peak on the horizontal frequency axis. The area under each peak can represent the quantity of the different metabolites. The phosphorus resonances from distinct phosphates on adenosine triphosphate (ATP) can thus be detected separately by ^{31}P MRS (Fig. 5). In order to detect such minute changes in NMR frequency caused by the chemical shift, an extremely homogeneous external magnetic field is necessary. The sharpness of each peak, or line width, is determined by the homogeneity of the magnetic field; increasing the homogeneity ('shimming') helps in obtaining narrow line widths[8]. In order to get an acceptable signal to noise ratio (SNR), the MR

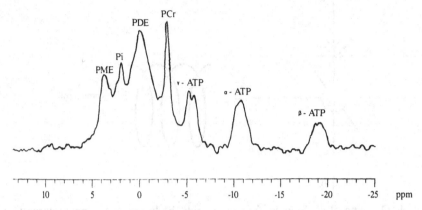

Fig. 5. The ³¹P NMR spectrum of a healthy human volunteer. (Reprinted from Keshavan et al., 1991, with permission by the American Psychiatric Association.)

signal has to be averaged many times; thus several minutes are needed to obtain a single MR spectrum. SNR is also affected by the rate at which the RF pulse is repeated (TR, or repetition time). When TR is shorter than T_1, saturation effects occur resulting in a reduction in signal.

For an element to be 'observable' by MRS, it should 1) have a magnetic spin and thus lend itself to 'excitation' by magnetic resonance; 2) be present in a detectable concentration (Table 1) and should produce an acceptable SNR; 3) be present in one or more biomolecules of interest; and 4) it must be technically feasible to obtain the MR signal from the region of interest. ³¹P, ¹H, ¹⁹F, ¹³C and ²³Na have to a varying extent met these conditions; using these elements it has been possible to study various aspects of metabolism.

Technical aspects of MRS

MRS essentially requires a magnet (including the gradient coils and shim coils), an RF transmitter and receiver coil tuned to the nucleus of interest, a display system and a computer (Fig. 6). Current spectrometers for human use operate from 1.5 to 4.0T. As opposed to MRI, MRS needs a higher magnetic field strength in order to preserve chemical shift information; a broad range of frequencies need to be generated to study nuclei with varying resonance frequencies. Further, the source of the signal needs to be localized to a volume of interest. The use of a surface coil placed near the area of interest is the simplest way to acquire signals from a subject[19]. Clinical applications of MRS have thus far mostly involved this technique (Fig. 7). The region of interest is usually limited in depth to one coil radius. The main disadvantage with surface coils is that volume selection is confined to a region near the surface.

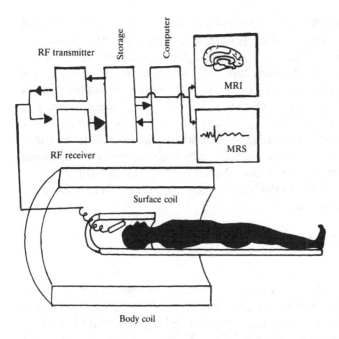

Fig. 6. Technical aspects of MRI and MRS: a schematic diagram.

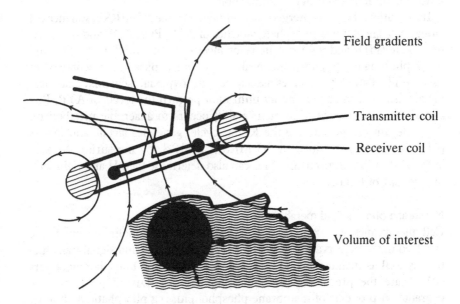

Fig. 7. Diagrammatic representation of a surface coil used for MRS. (Reprinted from Keshavan et al., 1991 with permission by the American Psychiatric Association.)

M S Keshavan and J W Pettegrew

There are several other approaches to localization, identified by a confusing array of acronyms, none of which is unanimously superior. Most involve an extension of MRI techniques, ie using magnetic gradients that make the frequency vary with the distance, thus enabling spatial encoding of the MR signal. These include the use of chemical shift imaging sequences (CSI)[11], depth resolved surface coil spectroscopy (DRESS)[20]; and image selected in vivo spectroscopy (ISIS)[21]. In CSI, 1, 2 or 3 dimensional spectral information can be obtained using a series of gradient fields. In the DRESS technique, a plane parallel to the face of a surface coil is selectively excited, and this results in spectral information from a disc shaped volume. Using ISIS the MRS signal can be localized to an axial 'slab', a column or a cube of brain tissue at a desired anatomical location.

Biochemical insights provided by MRS

Bioenergetics
Energy needed for living processes is generated by metabolism of carbo-hydrates, lipids and proteins, via the Krebs' cycle. This energy is secured as adenosine triphosphate (ATP); any excess is stored as phosphocreatine (PCr). PCr is catalysed by creative kinase (PCr + ADP → ATP + Creatine), and serves as an 'energy shuttle' which helps brain ATP levels to be constant. ATP is used for polymeric biosynthesis, structural repair, ion conduction, muscle contraction and nerve conduction.

Information about bioenergetics is contained in the ^{31}P MRS resonances of alpha, beta and gamma phosphate moieties of ATP, PCr, ADP and inorganic phosphate (Pi) α and γ phosphate resonances contain a mixture of ATP and other phosphates. β phosphate peaks represent a purer representation of tissue ATP. Pathological states associated with hypoxia, ischemia, anaerobic metabolism and impaired energy utilization perturb the levels of ATP, PCr and Pi. In the absence of oxygen, a shift occurs to anaerobic metabolism. Pyruvate, instead of entering the Krebs' cycle, generates lactate and lowers pH. Lactic acid is 'visible' by ^{1}H MRS; ^{31}P MRS, by measuring the acid induced shift in the spectrum of Pi, can also determine the pH and indirectly the amount of lactate.

Membrane phospholipid metabolism
Cell membranes are composed of a bilayer of phospholipids which are involved in the preservation of structure, ion conduction and signal transduc-tion as well as maintenance of concentration gradients. Phosphomonoesters (PME) are the precursors, and phosphodiesters (PDE) (Fig. 8) are the degradation products of membrane phospholipids, eg phosphatidyl choline, phosphatidyl ethanolamine and phosphatidyl serine[22]. Phosphomonoesters include phosphocholine, phosphoserine, phosphoethanolamine and α-gly-

Phospholipid metabolism

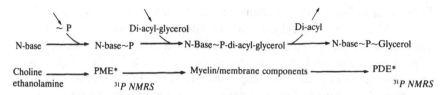

Fig. 8. A schematic diagram representing the major intermediates in phospholipid metabolism. Intermediates marked * are measurable using ^{31}P MRS. PME = phosphomonoester; PDE = phosphodiester; N-base = nitrogenous base.

cerophosphate; phosphodiesters include glycerophosphocholine and glycerophosphoethanolamine. Using ^{31}P MRS in vivo as well as in vitro studies of extracts of frozen brain tissue the concentration of the PME and PDEs and their ratios can be estimated; these measures reflect membrane turnover and may differ between health and disease states. Phospholipids, as well as mineral phosphates in bone constitute a large part of the broad resonance underlying the PDE and PME peaks.

Carbohydrate, amino acid and fat metabolism
In vivo ^{13}C-MRS can be used to measure and identify triglycerides, glycogen, and fats. Further definition can be obtained if a diet enriched in nonradioactive ^{13}C labelled-glucose or ^{13}C-acetate is fed. The signal obtained from this dose of ^{13}C can be used to study the way in which ingested nutrients are incorporated, stored and metabolized.

^{1}H MRS from tissue extracts reveals identifiable resonances from amino acids, neurotransmitters and their derivatives: metabolites related to energy metabolism such as glucose, phosphocreatine, creatine, lactate, and acetate and N-acetyl aspartate (NAA); metabolites related to phospholipid metabolism such as phosphocholine and phosphoethanolamine; and metabolites related to nucleotide metabolism such as adenine, guanine, uracil, and cytosine[23]. NAA is considered to be exclusively intraneuronal, and provides an index of neuronal mass and integrity. ^{1}H MRS, even though most sensitive, is limited by the intense background signal from ^{1}H in body water being 10 000 times more abundant than any other species, 'drowning' all other signals. Thus the water resonance and the resonances in the unprocessed ^{1}H MRS would appear like the mountain and a molehill placed side by side! However, computational techniques are available to 'suppress' the water resonance.

Electrolyte and PH measurement

^{23}Na, another element which lends itself to MRS, is largely extracellular. Disease states like injury, inflammation, edema and tissue death cause a shift of the ^{23}Na from extracellular to the intracellular compartment. Using paramagnetic shift reagents which are distributed exclusively in the extracellular compartment and shift the spectra from extracellular ^{23}Na signal, one can study the ratio of the two compartments. Thus, this technique may help in earlier identification of disease states affecting electrolyte balance.

An important aspect of the 'chemical shift' phenomenon is that the resonant frequencies of nuclei in relation to an acidic or basic group are sensitive to changes in pH. For example, the inorganic phosphate (Pi) can be used as a pH sensitive probe[24]. MRS is the only practical method available currently to measure in vivo pH in humans.

Neuropsychiatric applications

MRS as being applied to human disorders is relatively recent. The main areas where the clinical value of MRS appears established are in assessing the brain state, and estimating prognosis in neonates, and in detection of muscle enzyme defects. Its value in diagnosis and monitoring of neuropsychiatric disorders is far from being established. However, its value in research into the subcellular basis of neuropsychiatric disorders is obvious.

^{31}P MRS (Table 2)

^{31}P MRS has been the most widely applied technique because of the following advantages: 1) Since ^{31}P nucleus constitutes 100% of all phosphorus nuclei in the body, no labelling technique is required; 2) the ^{31}P nucleus provides sharp NMR signals for a variety of important phosphorus containing compounds; and 3) in vivo ^{31}P MRS analyses compare favourably with classic biochemical techniques without the need for tissue extraction.

Normal development and aging Membrane phospholipid and high energy phosphate metabolism are influenced considerably by brain development and aging, as demonstrated by high resolution ^{31}P MRS of rat brain extracts[22]. PCr and PDEs increase and PMEs decrease during dendritic proliferation and then remain stable till senescence. Similar findings have now been demonstrated by in vivo ^{31}P MRS in normal volunteers aged 8–86 years[25]. Healthy elderly subjects had decreased levels of PME, increased PDE, and decreased levels of nucleoside diphosphoderivatives such as UPD sugars and CDP choline or CDP ethanolamine. Thus MRS potentially provides in vivo biochemical information about normal aging process.

Dementias Through in vitro ^{31}P MRS studies of autopsy brain extracts from patients with Alzheimer's disease (AD), Pettegrew and colleagues have shown

Table 2. *³¹P MRS studies in neuropsychiatry*

	PME	PDE	Pi	PCr	ATP	pH
Alzheimer's disease	↑	↑	--	---	---	--
Schizophrenia	↓	↑	--	---	---	--
Autism	---	---	--	↑	↓	--
Epilepsy	---	---	--	---	---	↑
Aging	↓	↑	--	---	---	--
Development	↑	↑	--	---	---	--

an elevation in PME early in the disease followed by elevations in PDE as compared to nondiseased controls[26]. PME levels were inversely related and the PDE levels were positively related to the number of senile plaques. It was hypothesized that PME elevation occurs early in AD, and that PDE elevation occurs later paralleling the appearance of senile plaques. In vivo ³¹P MRS studies in AD patients have shown elevations of PME and of the ratio of PME to PDE in the temporoparietal regions, and elevations in Pi in the frontal and temporoparietal regions[27]. They also found that dementia severity scores were correlated negatively with PDE levels and positively with PCr levels[28]. These findings are different from the ³¹P MRS findings observed in association with normal aging, but are similar to the pattern seen during normal brain development. If confirmed, these in vivo ³¹P MRS findings could prove valuable in noninvasive monitoring of primary degenerative dementias.

Brown et al.[27] have shown elevations of PCr, and PCr/Pi ratios in 10 patients with Multiinfarct dementia (MID), as compared to patients with AD and age matched controls. This finding may reflect an impairment in energy mechanisms in MID. Values of the PCr/Pi ratios accurately classified 100% of the MID patients and 92% of the AD patients. PME and Pi also correctly classified all MID patients and all but one patient with AD. Thus, in vivo P MRS measurements are potentially valuable in the differential diagnosis between AD and MID. Some elevations in PDE levels have been detected in deeper tissues corresponding principally to white matter in two patients with Binswanger's disease, a disease of small vessels in the brain[29]. Significant elevations in PME and some elevations in PDE have also been reported in postmortem brain extracts from Huntington's chorea patients using ³¹P MRS[29].

HIV seropositive men have been reported to have significantly decreased ATP/Pi ratios; these changes were significantly correlated with the severity of neuropsychiatric impairment[30]. Bottomley et al.[31] have found significant decrements in PCr in AIDS dementia. Elevations in PME have also been seen in AIDS[32].

Neurodevelopmental disorders ^{31}P MRS studies in congenital cerebral atrophy, propionic acidemia, arginosuccinic acidemia, and meningitis in newborn infants have revealed decreased ratios of PCr/Pi and alterations in pH[17]. Such alterations predicted poor outcome and subsequent neurological abnormalities[33]. Minshew et al.[34] have recently compared the ^{31}P MRS profiles of 8 nondemented (ages 22–5 years; IQ 15–70) adult patients with Down's syndrome (DS) and eight age matched normal IQ controls. The DS patients had significantly increased PCr and decreased beta ATP; PME and PDE levels were not different.

Pettegrew et al.[35] have demonstrated that the autistics have decreased levels of PCr and of alpha ATP, suggesting alterations in brain high energy phosphate metabolism. These findings are distinct from those of schizophrenia, a condition for which autism can be frequently mistaken.

Epilepsies Seizures are associated with profound alterations in cerebral metabolism, and ^{31}P MRS provides an approach to monitor such changes in vivo. Schnall et al.[36] used triple nuclear MRS in vivo ([1]HP, ^{31}P, and [23]Na) during various levels of seizure activity in cats. They demonstrated increased lactate and decreased PCr during the seizures as well as an intracellular shift of the sodium ion pool. Weiner et al.[37] have shown an increase in pH and Pi in localized seizure foci in a patient with refractory complex partial seizures. The causal significance of these MRS findings to epilepsy are unclear.

Psychoses There is evidence suggesting that schizophrenia is associated with alterations in membrane phospholipids in peripheral cells[38], and this has stimulated studies of brain membrane composition using ^{31}P MRS. ^{31}P MRS studies of the prefrontal lobe have been carried out in neuroleptic naive first episode schizophrenics in comparison with age and sex matched controls[39,40]. The following metabolic alterations have been observed: 1) decreased PME levels; 2) increased PDE levels; 3) increased β-ATP levels; and 4) decreased levels of Pi. The PME and PDE results suggest decreased synthesis and increased breakdown of membrane phospholipids. Similar reduction in PME and increases in PDEs have been replicated in drug naive schizophrenics[41]. A similar pattern of decreased PME and increased PDE was seen in a 'normal' control who was studied 2 years before a psychotic episode, suggesting that these alterations may represent 'trait' markers[42]. The ^{31}P MRS findings appear to persist with neuroleptic treatment (Pettegrew et al., unpublished observations). The PDE levels correlate significantly with corpus callosal size, particularly with the anterior quartile[43]. O'Callaghan et al.[44] have carried out ^{31}P MRS in the left temporal lobe of 12 schizophrenic patients and 9 normal controls. No significant differences emerged, except for a higher pH in schizophrenic patients. However, the normal subjects were considerably older than schizophrenics and the effects of neuroleptics could not be excluded. Further, signal contributions from the temporali muscle could not be excluded. Williamson et al.[45] reported decreased PME but no change in PDE in chronic medicated schizophrenic patients compared to controls. They did not find any differences in β-ATP and Pi.

Pharmacological studies with ³¹P MRS ³¹P MRS studies can prove valuable in understanding the CNS effects of drugs, since they are noninvasive and can be repeated before and after administration of a pharmacological agent. Using ³¹P MRS, it is possible to detect accumulation of PMEs following lithium administration to cats in therapeutically meaningful doses[46]. It is an intriguing possibility that such effects could parallel lithium's therapeutic effects. ³¹P MRS studies have shown that calcium antagonists prevent the rapid decrease of ATP and PCr in rat brains during ischemia, indicating possibly a protective effect[47].

Using ³¹P MRS, one can noninvasively monitor second messenger mediated events in the living brain. ³¹P MRS has been used to detect the muscarinic agonist induced accumulation of phosphomonoesters (such as inositol phosphate) in cats[48]. It is thus possible to carry out longitudinal and drug related monitoring of changes in phospholipid metabolism in neuropsychiatric disorders. We have recently examined ³¹P MRS data in schizophrenic and schizoaffective patients before and after 1 and 2 weeks of treatment with lithium; reduced pretreatment PME and increases in nucleotide phosphates at 1 week predicted therapeutic response (Keshavan et al., unpublished observations).

¹⁹F MRS

The sensitivity of ¹⁹F is relatively high, making it attractive for MRS studies. ¹⁹F is the only naturally occurring fluorine isotope. Further, ¹⁹F has a large chemical shift range. There is very little mobile ¹⁹F in the body and it is biologically unimportant. ¹⁹F MRS has therefore been performed on artificially introduced biocompatible fluorocompounds, as in studies with blood substitutes[49], chemotherapeutic drugs, and fluorinated anesthetics. Recently, attempts have been made to determine concentrations of fluorinated neuroleptics such as fluphenazine[50,51]. In vivo ¹⁹F MRS has also been used to detect trifluoperazine and fluoxetine in brains of patients receiving these drugs[52]. The ability to spectroscopically localize the biodistribution of fluorinated psychotropic drugs might help in monitoring pharmacokinetics in vivo in the brain. Using fluorine labelled substrates such as 2-fluoro-2-deoxy glucose it has been possible to follow glucose metabolism in rats[53]. ¹⁹ MRS has also been used to measure cerebral blood flow[54]. With future developments in MRS technology it should be possible to measure fluorinated neurotransmitter ligands in the human brain.

^{13}C MRS

98.9% of naturally abundant carbon is ^{12}C, and is not detectable by MRS. The 1.1% natural abundance ^{13}C resonances are 'visible' in extracts. Natural abundance ^{13}C MRS of rat brain demonstrates ^{13}C chemical shifts of brain metabolites and contains significant information about amino acid and neurotransmitter levels (glutamate, γ-aminobutyrate) and some information about phospholipid and energy metabolism. The main limitation of natural abundance ^{13}C MRS is in poor sensitivity.

^{13}C labelled substrates such as glucose have proved to be an elegant method to study selected areas of metabolism in vivo and in vitro. Hammer et al.[55] have localized ^{13}C glucose signals in monkey brain and were able to follow metabolism serially following intravenous ^{13}C glucose administration. The advantage of the labelled ^{13}C-MRS studies is that metabolites of the parent compound are simultaneously detected, allowing successive steps in metabolism to be analysed in physiological states and diseases.

^{1}H MRS (Table 3)

In vivo application of ^{1}H MRS has had a relatively late start. The limitations of ^{1}H MRS include 1) the relatively narrow range of 'visible' chemical shifts (10 ppm) compared to ^{31}P MRS (40 ppm); 2) the diversity of proton containing molecules in living tissues; and 3) the dominant water signal of most biological systems. Despite these limitations several findings of interest have emerged from ^{1}H MRS research:

Neurological disorders ^{1}H MRS has revealed cerebral lactate elevation in clinical epilepsy[56]. ^{1}H and ^{31}P MRS in patients with hepatic encephalopathy have revealed increases in glutamine and phosphocholine and a decrease in choline[57]. Using ^{1}H MRS, decreases in N-acetyl aspartate (NAA)[58] have been found in patients with cerebrovascular disease. Significant changes also have been observed in multiple sclerosis[59]. Using in vitro ^{1}H MRS, Klunk et al.[60] have demonstrated decreased NAA and increased glutamate in brains of patients with Alzheimer's disease. The decrease in NAA correlated with the number of senile plaques and neurofibrillary tangles. The decreases in NAA might reflect neuronal loss; the remaining neurones may thus be exposed to relatively high levels of glutamate, perhaps leading to neurotoxic brain damage. These exciting findings need to be examined by in vivo ^{1}H MRS.

Psychoses Sharma et al.[61] have obtained ^{1}H spectra from the frontal and occipital regions of 9 psychiatric patients and 9 healthy controls: the patients, notably lithium treated bipolar disorders, showed an increased NAA/PCr ratio compared to controls. Charles et al.[62] have recently observed a trend for increased choline among elderly depressives; these levels subsided following treatment. Stanley et al. 1992 have compared ^{1}H MRS data from never

Table 3. *^{1}H MRS studies in neuropsychiatry*

	Lactate	NAA	Choline	Glutamate
Schizophrenia	-------	↓	-------	↓
Depression	-------	---	↑	---------
Epilepsy	↑	---	-------	---------
Multiplesclerosis	-------	↓	-------	
Stroke	-------	↓	-------	---------

treated schizophrenics with controls and have found significantly reduced glutamate mole % in the schizophrenics in the dorsolateral prefrontal cortex[63]. Further studies are needed to explore this interesting observation. Nasrallah et al.[64] have conducted ^{1}H MRS studies of the hippocampus in schizophrenic. They show a decrement in NAA in the right hippocampus; they interpret this deficit as reflecting possible neuronal loss.

Electroconvulsive therapy Localized ^{1}H spectroscopy has been used to monitor brain metabolism following electroconvulsive therapy[65]. An increase was seen in the lipid resonance; the authors speculated that this may be related to maximal activation of the phosphoinositide system.

Other psychiatric disorders Proton spectroscopy is of potential value in research into panic disorders. Lactate infusion, known to induce panic attacks, produces a consistent and detectable elevation in brain lactate[66]. In vivo proton MRS has also been applied to alcoholism research. A ^{1}H MRS study showed that alcohol resulted in increased CNS membrane fluidity and high water content of tissues in rats[67]. The methylproton signal of alcohol can be observed in the human brain using ^{1}H MRS at levels of legal intoxication (0.1%)[68]. This approach can be used to study regional distribution and kinetics of ethanol.

Brain development ^{1}H MRS has also provided valuable information about neonatal brain development. Elevations of choline have been attributed to myelination; increases in N-acetyl aspartate are also associated with neuronal development[69].

Activation studies Physiological activation studies have been conducted using ^{1}H MRS. An alteration in lactate has been observed following auditory stimulation in the temporal lobes[70].

^{23}Na MRS

Even though ^{23}Na is 100% naturally abundant, it gives rise to very broad peaks due to its rapid T_2 relaxation, making it a poor choice for MRS. Only 40% of the intracellular sodium is 'visible' by MR spectroscopy when the cell membranes are intact[71]. Further, Na^+ does not form covalent bonds with other atoms, and therefore, chemical shift information is not obtainable. Sodium exists within aqueous macromolecular complexes both inside and outside the cell; membrane impermeable paramagnetic agents such as dysprosium polyphosphate can selectively alter the extracellular ^{23}Na chemical shift and thus can allow the resolution of the extra and intracellular pools into distinct resonances. Dysprosium tripolyphosphate, used for the above purpose in animal and tissue studies, has not been used in humans for reasons of toxicity.

^{23}Na MRS has been applied to study disorders involving sodium transport and membrane disruption. ^{23}Na MRS without shift reagents in human studies shows dramatically elevated ^{23}Na in stroke, hemorrhage and brain tumours[72].

^{7}Li-MRS

^{7}Li MRS could be a valuable approach to the intracellular chemistry of lithium. An in vitro ^{7}Li-MRS study has provided evidence that lithium increases molecular motion by interaction with the membrane associated cytoskeleton in human erythrocytes[73]. In vivo ^{7}Li NMR studies have recently been carried out in humans[74-76]. In the latter two studies, the brain lithium levels as measured by ^{7}Li MRS correlated well with serum levels. Based on their data, Guilai et al.[75] suggested that the minimum effective brain concentration of lithium for maintenance therapy in bipolar disorder is around 0.2–0.3 meq/l.

Advantages of MRS

Until very recently, only indirect methods such as examination of blood, urine, cerebrospinal fluid and autopsy brain, were available to investigate brain chemistry. The advent of physiological imaging techniques therefore represent a major advance. MRS has several unique advantages. It is noninvasive and is therefore ideal for longitudinal studies; there is no established evidence that magnetic fields cause harm, though possible long-term risks have not been fully evaluated. MRS provides information about intracellular pH as well as the motion of molecules and their quantitation not available by other techniques; one can examine metabolic turnover directly, and can be expressed as mole %, the important unit that controls chemical reactions and which is not affected by partial volume effects. A large number of chemicals including metabolics and drugs are potentially amenable to quantification.

Limitations of MRS

Several disadvantages have hindered progress in the application of MRS in clinical medicine. Many of them are technical; others are patient related[18].

Technical limitations

1. MRS requires magnetic fields to be stronger and more homogeneous, and also needs 'shimming' for each measurement making it more expensive in time and cost. Because the MRS signals are much weaker than the proton signals used for MRI, signal acquisition needs more time, and the volume of interest has to be much larger than that for MRI.
2. Not all elements can be studied by MRS. The intrinsic sensitivity (ability of an element to resonate), of elements such as ^{39}K being very low make them inaccessible to MRS. Further, certain elements with high sensitivity such as ^{19}F are present in the body in very low concentrations so that they cannot be used in MRS studies in their natural state. The 'overall sensitivity' of a given nucleus is its intrinsic sensitivity multiplied by its concentration in the tissue. In any given volume of interest, the current limit of detection is about 10^{-6} that of water protons.
3. Only highly mobile nuclei which are in solution, are MRS 'visible'. Nuclei whose mobility is restricted because of binding to membranes or macromolecules result in broad resonance signals with poor signal to noise ratio. For this reason, only a few selected aspects of metabolism can be studied by MRS.
4. The prolonged acquisition time limits detection of transient biochemical changes. For this reason, MRS cannot yet be adequately applied in cognitive or neurophysiological challenge paradigms.
5. NMR machines are quite expensive. This raises the important question of whether MRS is cost-effective, and whether the information provided is clinically useful.

Subject-related limitations

Several subject related variables also need to be considered in interpreting MRS studies.

1. *Subject cooperation.* Subject cooperation is a key factor, and is often limited in psychiatric patients. Claustrophobia can be a particularly difficult problem; in about 1% of subjects, NMR studies fail because of this problem.
2. *Motion artefacts.* Random patient motion, as well as involuntary motion caused by blood or CSF flow, respiration, and peristalsis could affect the quality of spectra in MRS. Using complex gradients, it is possible to suppress motion artefacts.
3. *Partial volume effects.* Biochemical information provided by MRS usually conforms to geometrically shaped volumes, eg spherical, and not to

the shapes of anatomical structures of interest to the psychiatrist. Further, signals 'bleed' from one voxel to another, leading to blurring of voxel edges. Regional differences in brain structure, eg superficial versus deeper structures could also affect the interpretability of MRS data.

MRS and other 'functional' imaging techniques

Positron emission tomography (PET) and single photon emission tomography (SPECT) scans provide alternative, promising approaches to functional brain imaging (Table 4). The advantages of PET scanning include relatively high sensitivity, high spatial resolution, and the feasibility of investigating a wide range of biochemical processes including glucose and oxygen consumption, neurotransmitter turnover and neuroreceptor binding. The disadvantages include the use of radioactive tracers with its attendant risks, and the need for an expensive cyclotron nearby to make such isotopes. SPECT scanning offers the advantage of not requiring such expensive facility and can potentially provide information about a wide range of biochemical processes, but has a relatively low resolution. Thus it can be seen that PET and SPECT scanning have advantages not seen with MRS; MRS likewise has unique advantages. These techniques may therefore be complementary, and are likely to represent competitors among the developing brain imaging technologies.

Recently, a novel approach to functional brain imaging has been developed using principles of NMR. This involves quantitative imaging of brain hemodynamics using the principle of echo-planar imaging and using an intravenous paramagnetic agent, gadolinum. This technique has been used to acquire images of regional cerebral blood flow during activation and resting states[77]. This approach enjoys excellent temporal resolution, and in this regard is clearly superior to PET.

Future developments

Clinical research application of MRS has so far mainly involved ^{31}P studies. In view of the relatively high NMR sensitivities, the ^{1}H metabolites such as neurotransmitters and amino acids are promising avenues for future research in clinical applications of MRS. Newer techniques of suppressing signals from water and fat are likely to make this approach more feasible. ^{13}C and ^{23}Na MRS represent other noninvasive techniques for viewing brain chemistry. ^{7}Li and ^{19}F MRS will offer new ways to study the kinetics and function of psychopharmacological agents. Most MRS studies are now done with magnets of 1.5 to 2.5T. However, instruments of 4.0T are now being used, and dual-purpose MRI/MRS instruments are available. Future clinical applications also will benefit from the use of spectroscopy contrast agents which enhance chemical shift. It is already possible to incorporate MRS data into an image, much like the PET scan (spectroscopic imaging). Spatial resolutions

Table 4. *Physiological imaging techniques: relative merits*

	PET	SPECT	MRS
Spatial resolution	+++	++	+
Temporal resolution	+++	++	+
Cost	+++	+	++
Safety	+	++	+++
Sensitivity	+++	++	+

of about 1 cm^3 have been achieved. Three dimensional phase encoding is now possible, allowing mapping of proton metabolites in all three spatial dimensions of the human brain[78]. 'Metabolic maps' of the brain can be developed by simultaneous use of multinuclear spectroscopic techniques in vivo, eg using ^{31}P nuclei for ATP and ^{1}H for lactate. The technologies of MRI and MRS are increasingly converging to yield spatial chemical images providing novel opportunities for clinical research. Recently, there has also been increasing interest in solid state NMR studies of brain tissue[7] and NMR microscopy, with which it is possible to identify intracellular structures[79]. Both these approaches may eventually be applied in clinical research settings.

While the prospects are promising, the potential clinical applications of MRS in the psychiatric setting are still far away, and more needs to be learned. Future research in neuropsychiatric MRS will be guided by the following goals: a) examining specificity of MRS findings in carefully selected patients with major neuropsychiatric disorders and appropriate controls; b) reexamining in vivo information from patients in the light of modern neurochemistry; c) exploring structure–function relationships by simultaneous use of MRI and MRS; d) conducting MRS studies in different brain areas relevant to pathophysiology of neuropsychiatric disorder, such as limbic areas and temporal lobes; and e) studying biochemical parameters to delineate treatment effects, predictors of treatment response, identify biological correlates of course of illness and to develop novel treatment strategies.

The field of neuropsychiatric MRS is still in its infancy. It has been stated recently that it is the analytical method of the twenty first century[80]. Much of the research so far has involved 'fishing expeditions' in 'uncharted waters'[1]. Focused and careful research is, however, likely to yield rich dividends for psychiatry whose disorders still remain poorly understood.

Acknowledgements

Supported in part by Scottish Rite Schizophrenia Foundation Grant No. 5–37100 (MS Keshavan). We are grateful to Sharon Stephenson for secretarial help.

M S Keshavan and J W Pettegrew

References

(1) Lock T, Abou-saleh MT, Edwards RHT. Psychiatry and the new magnetic resonance era. *Br J Psychiat* 1990; 157(Suppl 9): 38–55.
(2) Pettegrew JW, ed. *NMR: principles and applications to biomedical research.* New York: Springer-Verlag, 1990.
(3) Andrew ER, Bydder G, Griffiths J, Iles R, Styles P. *Clinical magnetic resonance imaging and spectroscopy.* New York: John Wiley and Son, 1990.
(4) Cady EB. *Clinical magnetic resonance spectroscopy.* New York: Plenum Press, 1990.
(5) Keshavan MS, Kapur S, Pettegrew JW. magnetic resonance spectroscopy: potential, pitfalls and promise. *Am J Psychiat* 1991; 148: 976–85.
(6) Bottomley PA. Human in vivo NMR spectroscopy in diagnostic medicine: clinical tool or research probe? *Radiology* 1989; 170: 1–15.
(7) Weiner MW. The promise of magnetic resonance spectroscopy for medical diagnosis. *Invest Radiol* 1988; 23: 253–61.
(8) Pettegrew JW. Nuclear magnetic resonance: principles and applications to neuroscience research. In: Boller F, Grafman J, eds. *Handbook of neuropsychology,* vol 5. Amsterdam: Elsevier, 1991: 35–56.
(9) Andreasen NC. Nuclear magnetic resonance imaging. In: Andreasen NC, ed. *Brain imaging: applications in psychiatry.* American Psychiatric Press, 1989: 67–123.
(10) Becker ED, Fisk CL. NMR: physical principles and current status as a biomedical technique. *Ann NY Acad Sci* 1987; 508: 1–9.
(11) Pykett IL, Rosen BR. Nuclear magnetic resonance in vivo proton chemical shift imaging. *Radiology* 1983; 149: 197–201.
(12) Purcell EM, Torrey HC, Pound RV. Resonance absorption by nuclear magnetic movements in a solid. *Phys Rev* 1946; 69: 37–8.
(13) Bloch R, Hansen WW, Packard ME. Nuclear induction. *Phys Rev* 1946; 69: 127.
(14) Andrew ER. A historical review of NMR and its clinical applications. *Br Med Bull* 1984; 40: 2, 115–19.
(15) Moon RB, Richards JH. Determination of intracellular pH by ^{31}P magnetic resonance. *J Biol Chem* 1973; 248: 7276–8.
(16) Hoult DI, Busby SJW, Gadian DG. Observation of tissue metabolites using ^{31}P nuclear magnetic resonance. *Nature* 1974; 252: 285–7.
(17) Cady EB, Costello AM, Dawson MJ et al. Noninvasive investigation of cerebral metabolism in newborn infants by phosphorus nuclear magnetic resonance spectroscopy. *Lancet* 1983; i: 1059–62.
(18) Lauterbur PC. Image formation by induced local interactions: examples employing nuclear magnetic resonance. *Nature* 1973; 242: 190–1.
(19) Ackerman JJH, Grove TH, Wong GG et al. Mapping of metabolites in whole animals by ^{31}P NMR using surface coils. *Nature* 1980; 283: 167–70.
(20) Bottomley PA, Foster TH, Darrow RD. Depth resolved surface coil spectroscopy (DRESS) for in vivo ^{1}H, ^{31}P, and ^{31}C NMR. *J Mag Reson* 1984; 59: 338–42.
(21) Ordidge RJ, Connelly A, Lohman JAB. Image-selected in vivo spectroscopy

(ISIS) a new technique for spatially selective NMR spectroscopy. *J Mag Reson* 1986; 66: 283–94.

(22) Pettegrew JW, Panchalingam K, Withers G et al. Changes in brain energy and phospholipid metabolism during development and aging in the Fischer 344 rat. *J Neuropath Exp Neurol* 1990; 49: 237–49.

(23) Luyten PR, Hollander JA. Observation of metabolites in the human brain by MR spectroscopy. *Radiology* 1986; 161: 795–8.

(24) Pettegrew JW, Withers G, Panchalingam K et al. Considerations for brain pH assessment by ^{31}P NMR. *Mag Res Imaging* 1988; 6: 135–42.

(25) Panchalingam K, Pettegrew JW, Strychor S, Tretta M. Effect of normal aging on membrane phospholipid metabolism by ^{31}P in vivo NMR spectroscopy [Abstract]. *Soc Neurosci* 1990; 16: 843.

(26) Pettegrew JW, Panchalingam K, Moossy J et al. Correlation of ^{P} magnetic resonance spectroscopy and morphological findings in Alzheimer's disease. *Arch Neurol* 1988; 45(10): 1093–6.

(27) Brown GG, Levin SR, Gorrell JM et al. In vivo ^{31}P NMR profiles of Alzheimer's disease and multiple subcortical infarct dementia. *Neurology* 1989; 39: 1423–7.

(28) Pettegrew JW, Panchalingam K, Huff J et al. Metabolic alterations in the dorsolateral prefrontal cortex of Alzheimer's disease [Abstract]. *Book of abstracts of the eighth annual meeting of the Society of Magnetic Resonance in Medicine*. Berkeley, California, 1989.

(29) Smith LS, Bottomley PA, Drayer BP et al. Localized clinical ^{31}P NMR spectroscopy in Huntington's, Parkinsons', Alzheimer's and Binswanger's diseases [Abstract]. *Book of abstracts of the Society of Magnetic Resonance in Medicine*. Berkeley, California, 1986.

(30) Deicken R, Hubesch B, Jensen P et al. Alterations in brain phosphate metabolite concentrations in patients with HIV infection. *Arch Neurol* 1990; 48: 203–9.

(31) Bottomley PA, Hardy CJ, Cousins JP et al. HIV dementia complex: brain high energy phosphate metabolism. *Neuroradiology* 1990; 176: 407–41.

(32) Cadoux-Hudsen J, Rajagopalan B, Radda GK et al. Metabolic changes due to HIV infection in human brain in vivo. *Mag Reson Med* 1990; 2: 991.

(33) Hamilton PA, Hope PL, Cady EB et al. Impaired energy metabolism in brains of newborn infants with increased cerebral echodensities. *Lancet* 1986; i: 1242–6.

(34) Minshew NJ, Pettegrew JW, Panchalingam K. Membrane phospholipid alterations in Alzheimer's disease are not present in Down's syndrome [Abstract]. *Biol Psychiat* 1990; 27(9a): 41–42.

(35) Pettegrew JW, Minshew NJ, Payton JB. ^{31}P NMR in normal IQ adult autistics [Abstract]. *Biol Psychiat* 1989; 25 (Suppl): 182–3.

(36) Schnall MD, Yoshizakik, Chance B et al. Triple nuclear NMR studies of cerebral metabolism during generalized seizure. *Mag Reson Med* 1988; 6: 15–23.

(37) Weiner MW, Hetherington H, Hubetsch B et al. Clinical magnetic resonance spectroscopy of brain, heart, liver, kidney and cancer. *NMR Biomed* 1989; 2: 290–7.

(38) Rotrosen J, Wolkin A. Phospholipid and protaglandin hypothesis of schizophrenia. In: Meltzer HY, ed. *Psychopharmacology the third generation of progress*. New York: Raven Press, 1987: 759–65.

(39) Pettegrew JW, Keshavan M, Panchalingam K et al. Alterations in brain high energy phosphate and membrane phospholipid metabolism in first episode, drug naive schizophrenics. *Arch Gen Psychiat* 1991; 48: 563–8.

(40) Keshavan MS, Pettegrew JW, Panchalingam K et al. In vivo ^{31}P MRS of the frontal lobe in neuroleptic naive first episode psychosis: preliminary observations. *Schizophrenia Res* 1989; 2: 123.

(41) Stanley JA, Williamson P, Drost DJ, Carr T, Morrison S, Merskey H. Membrane phospholipid metabolism abnormalities in the left prefrontal cortex in drug-naive and chronic schizophrenics via ^{31}P NMR spectroscopy. In: *Works in progress, Society of Magnetic Resonance in Medicine, tenth annual scientific meeting*. San Francisco: 1991; 1062.

(42) Keshavan MS, Pettegrew JW, Panchalingam K et al. [31]P magnetic resonance spectroscopy detects altered membrane metabolism before onset of schizophrenia. *Arch Gen Psychiat* 1991; 48: 1112–13.

(43) Sanders RD, Keshavan MS, Pettegrew JW et al. Frontal lobe metabolism and cerebral morphology in schizophrenia. *Schizophrenia Res* 1992; (in press).

(44) O'Callaghan E, Redmond O, Ennis R et al. Initial investigation of the left temporo parietal region in schizophrenia by ^{31}P magnetic resonance spectroscopy. *Biol Psychiat* 1991; 29: 1149–52.

(45) Williamson P, Drost D, Stanley J et al. Localized phosphorus [31] magnetic resonance spectroscopy in chronic schizophrenic patients and normal controls. *Arch Gen Psychiat* 1991; 48: 578.

(46) Renshaw PF, Summer JJ, Renshaw CE et al. Changes in the ^{31}P NMR spectra of cats receiving lithium chloride systemically. *Biol Psychiat* 1986; 21: 691–4.

(47) Sauter A, Rudin M. Effects of calcium agonists on high energy phosphates in ischemic rat brain measured by ^{31}P NMR spectroscopy. *Mag Reson Med* 1987; 4: 1–8.

(48) Renshaw PS, Schnall MD, Leigh JS. In vivo ^{31}P NMR spectroscopy of agonist stimulated phosphatidylinositol metabolism in cat brain. *Mag Reson Med* 1987; 4: 221–6.

(49) Joseph PM, Yuasa Y, Kundel HL et al. Magnetic resonance imaging of fluorine in rats infused with artificial blood. *Invest Radiol* 1985; 20: 504–9.

(50) Bartels M, Albert K, Kruppa G et al. Fluorinated psychopharmacological agents, noninvasive observation by fluorine 19 nuclear magnetic resonance. *Psychiat Res* 18: 197–201.

(51) Arndt BC, Ratner AW, Faull KS et al. [19]F magnetic resonance imaging spectroscopy of a fluorinated neuroleptic ligand; in vitro and *in vivo* studies. *Psychiat Res* 1988; 25: 73–9.

(52) Komorowski RA, Newton JED, Karson C et al. Detection of psychoactive drugs in vivo humans using ^{19}F NMR spectroscopy. *Biol Psychiat* 1990; 29: 711–14.

(53) Berkowitz BA, Ackerman JJH. 2-fluoro-2-deoxy D glucose (FDG) metabolism in vivo: a ^{19}F-[^{1}H] NMR study [Abstract]. *Book of Abstracts of the Society of Magnetic Resonance in Medicine* 1985; 1: 759–60.

(54) Bolas NM, Petros AJ, Bergel D et al. Use of ^{19}F magnetic resonance spec-

troscopy for measurement of cerebral blood flow [Abstract]. *Book of Abstracts of the Society of Magnetic Resonance in Medicine* 1985; 1: 315–16.

(55) Hammer BE, Sacks W, Hennessy MJ et al. Investigations of in vivo glucose metabolism by C-13 MR imaging. *Radiology* 1985; 157(P): 220.

(56) Matthews PM, Arnold DL. In vivo proton magnetic resonance spectroscopy in the study of focal epilepsy in man [Abstract]. *Book of Abstracts of the Society of Magnetic Resonance in Medicine eighth annual meeting* 1989; 1: 371.

(57) Kreis R, Farrow N, Ross BD. Diagnosis of hepatic encephalopathy by proton magnetic resonance spectroscopy. *Lancet* 1990; 336: 635–6.

(58) Bruhm H, Frahm J, Gyngell ML et al. Cerebral metabolism in man after acute stroke: new observations using localized proton nuclear magnetic resonance spectroscopy. *Mag Reson Med* 1989; 9: 126–31.

(59) Arnold DL, Matthews PM, Francis G et al. Proton magnetic resonance spectroscopy of human brain in vivo in the evaluation of multiple sclerosis: assessments of the load of the disease. *Mag Reson Med* 1990; 14: 154–9.

(60) Klunk WE, Panchalingam K, Moossy J et al. N-acetyl-L-aspartate and other aminoacid metabolites in Alzheimer's disease brain: a preliminary proton magnetic resonance study. *Neurology*; (in press).

(61) Sharma RP, Subramanian PNV, Barany et al. Proton magnetic resonance spectroscopy of the brain. *New Research Program and Abstracts, American Psychiatric Association 143rd annual meeting*. Washington: 1990: 71.

(62) Charles HC, Lazeyras F, Krishnan R et al. Brain choline in depression: in vivo detection of potential pharmacodynamic effects of antidepressant therapy using hydrogen localized spectroscopy. *Biol Psychiat*; (in press).

(63) Stanley JA, Williamson PC, Drost DJ et al. In vivo proton magnetic resonance spectroscopy in never treated schizophrenics. *New Research Abstract NR10*. Washington: American Psychiatric Association, 1992.

(64) Nasrallah HA, Skinner TE, Schmaibrook PE et al. In vivo ^{1}H NMR spectroscopy of the hippocampus in schizophrenia [Abstract]. *ACNP 30th meeting*, Puerto Rico, 1991: 19.

(65) Woods BT, Chiu TM. In vivo ^{1}H spectroscopy of the human brain following electroconvulsive therapy. *Ann Neurol* 1990; 28: 745–9.

(66) Dager SR, Marro KI, Metzger G et al. Detection of whole brain lactate increases during intravenous 1 M sodium L-lactate infusion by NMR spectroscopy. In: *Works in Progress, Society of Magnetic Resonance in Medicine, tenth annual scientific meeting*. San Francisco, 1991: 1048.

(67) Besson JAO, Greentree SG, Foster MA et al. Effects of ethanol on the NMR characteristics of rat brain. *Br J Psychiat* 1989; 155: 818–21.

(68) Hanstock CC, Rothman DL, Shulman RG et al. Measurement of ethanol in the human brain using NMR spectroscopy. *J Stud Alcohol* 1990; 51: 104–7.

(69) Kreis R, Ernst T, Arcinue E et al. Mo-Inositol in short TE ^{1}H-MRS: a new indicator of neonatal brain development and pathology. In: *Works in Progress, Society of Magnetic Resonance in Medicine, tenth annual scientific meeting*. San Francisco, 1991: 1007.

(70) Singh M, Brechner RR, Terk MR et al. Increased lactate in the stimulated human auditory cortex. In: *Works in Progress, Society of Magnetic Resonance in Medicine, tenth annual scientific meeting*. San Francisco, 1991: 1008.

(71) Cope FW. NMR evidence for complexing of Na$^+$ in muscle, kidney and brain,

and by actomyosin. The relation of cellular complexing of Na$^+$ to water structure and to transport kinetics. *J Gen Physiol* 1967; 50: 1353–75.
(72) Hilal SK, Maudsley AA, Raj B et al. In vivo NMR imaging of sodium-23 in the human head. *J Comput Assist Tomogr* 1985; 9: 1–7.
(73) Pettegrew JW, Short JW, Woessner RD et al. The effect of lithium on the membrane molecular dynamics of normal human erythrocytes. *Biol Psychiat* 1987; 22: 857–71.
(74) Newton J, Komoroski R, Walker E et al. Lithium-7 NMR spectroscopy of human brain [Abstract]. *Biol Psychiat* 1989; 25: 136.
(75) Gyulai L, Wicklund SW, Greenstein R et al. Measurement of tissue lithium concentration by lithium magnetic resonance spectroscopy in patients with disorder. *Biol Psychiat* 1991; 29: 1161–70.
(76) Renshaw PF, Haselgrove JC, Leigh JS et al. In vivo nuclear magnetic resonance imaging of lithium. *Mag Reson Med* 1985; 2: 512–16.
(77) Belliveau JW, Kennedy JN, McKinstry RC et al. Functional mapping of the human visual cortex by magnetic resonance imaging. *Science* 1991; 254: 716–18.
(78) Duyn JH, Matson GB, Weiner MW. 3D phase encoding methods for ^{1}H spectroscopic imaging of human brain. In: *Works in progress, Society of Magnetic Resonance in Medicine, tenth annual scientific meeting.* San Francisco: 1991: 1005.
(79) Aguayo J, Blackband S, Schoeninger J et al. Nuclear magnetic resonance imaging of a single cell. *Nature* 1986; 322: 190–1.
(80) Vine W. Clinical diagnosis by nuclear magnetic resonance spectroscopy. *Arch Pathol Lab Med* 1990; 114: 453–62.

Index

Index